Also by David Abrahamsen

Crime and the Human Mind

Men, Mind and Power

The Mind and Death of a Genius

Report on a Study of 102 Sex Offenders at Sing
    Sing Prison as Submitted to Governor Thomas E.
    Dewey

Who are the Guilty? A Study of Education and
    Crime

The Road to Emotional Maturity

The Psychology of Crime

The Emotional Care of Your Child

Our Violent Society

The Murdering Mind

Nixon vs. Nixon: An Emotional Tragedy

THE
MIND OF THE
ACCUSED

A Psychiatrist
in the Courtroom

DAVID ABRAHAMSEN, M.D.

SIMON AND SCHUSTER
New York

Published by Simon and Schuster
A Division of Simon & Schuster, Inc.
Simon & Schuster Building
Rockefeller Center
1230 Avenue of the Americas
New York, New York 10020
SIMON AND SCHUSTER and colophon are registered trademarks of Simon &
Schuster, Inc.
Designed by C. Linda Dingler
Manufactured in the United States of America

10 9 8 7 6 5 4 3 2 1

Library of Congress Cataloging in Publication Data

Abrahamsen, David, date.
    The mind of the accused.

    Includes bibliographical references and index.
    1. Insanity—Jurisprudence—United States. 2. Criminal liability—United
States. 3. Forensic psychiatry—United States.   I. Title
KF9242.A72   1983   345.73'04   83-16176
ISBN 0-671-47053-1   347.3054

ACKNOWLEDGMENTS

I thank Don Congdon, my literary agent, who years ago encouraged me to write a book about my psychiatric patients and criminal cases; Helga Moor, my secretary, for her perspicacity in deciphering my handwritten drafts and for editorial suggestions; Gene Brown, for his contribution to the writing of the manuscript; Fred Hills, Senior Editor at Simon and Schuster, for his constructive and stimulating suggestions.

I am grateful to *The New York Times*, in particular A. M. Rosenthal, Executive Editor, for securing sources that concern my findings.

Warm thanks go to my wife, Lova, who has played an integral role in the writing of this book, and who with courage has shared with me the many events a writer and a psychoanalyst experiences.

D.A.

To Kari, Peter, Alec,
Jeremy and Molly

CONTENTS

PREFACE

For nearly a half-century, the mind of the accused and the issue of criminal responsibility have been central concerns of my career as Freudian psychoanalyst and forensic psychiatrist. This book draws on cases from my own experience to illustrate how we must unravel the complexities of the mind, both criminal and innocent, before we can fairly establish guilt and justify criminal penalties. In each case I've tried to show *why* a person behaved as he did, not merely where he should be classified on the broad spectrum from normal to psychotic.

In a sense, these are detective stories. The reader will see how a forensic psychiatrist deals with all the unknown factors in a criminal case; how true symptoms are distinguished from spurious, and actual motivation from mere acting. In that respect the working of the psychiatrist's mind is very important; therefore, I have given some account of how I came to this strange and challenging field, and of the theory and methods I use to get to the bottom of a case.

In the past decade, the question of the insanity plea in particular has become increasingly controversial; in fact, many people feel that criminals are able to literally get away with murder these days by pleading insanity. Not-guilty verdicts in several recent, well-publicized trials, such as that of John Hinckley, would-be assassin of President Reagan, have increased opposition to the use of the insanity plea. Lay persons, as well as legal and psychiatric professionals, have been appalled at the spectacle of the defense pitting the testimony of its psychiatric experts against those speaking for the prosecution, each attributing to the defendant a different set of conscious and unconscious motivations, all of which are described in esoteric, multisyllabic psychological jargon.

I have observed and participated in a great deal of courtroom drama as an expert witness, both for the prosecution and for the defense. My testimony has sent murderers feigning insanity, such as David Berkowitz (the Son of Sam killer), to prison, and the truly criminally insane, such as George Metesky (the Mad Bomber), to psychiatric hospitals.

The use of psychiatric testimony in court will always be problematic, its subjectivity rooted in the nature of the mind and human behavior. But it need not be arbitrary, and if the relevant laws are clearly understood and carefully applied, a fair and acceptable verdict can be expected. In describing those laws and showing how they have been used—and abused—in a variety of cases, I hope to scatter some of the clouds that envelop the concept of criminal insanity and demonstrate the continuing value of the age-old distinction between act and intent.

1
LIFE V. DEATH

When the call came late that night, the connection was bad, and I could not determine what was the matter with the patient—only that I should come immediately. It was not unusual for a public-health physician in Norway in the 1930s to be called out on emergencies, and I knew that a long slow ride through the countryside lay ahead. I grabbed my medicine bag and flashlight and drove up from the valley where I was stationed to meet the horse and buggy that would take me the rest of the way.

In the dark I could see almost nothing except the vague outline of the horse's rump moving in front of me and the driver to my left. I turned on my flashlight to explore the darkness and was horrified to see the edge of a deep ravine right next to me, falling away from the road into darkness. At last the path broadened into something that passed for a road. Soon we came to a group of houses where a man who had been awaiting my arrival made signs to me to follow him. I assumed he was going to take me to one of the houses; but instead he led me to a barn. There must have been some mistake.

"I'm not a veterinarian," I told him, but he only looked at me grimly. He opened a large door that creaked on its hinges and we entered the gloomy interior, redolent of hay and cows. I shined my flashlight around, still wondering what I had been summoned for. There were no animals. Then, high up, the light caught something. The body of a man was hanging by the neck from one of the rafters.

When we finally cut him down, I could see that the dead man had been about thirty—only two years older than I was then. Why had he killed himself? Could he have been helped? For him it no longer mattered, but I couldn't stop thinking about it. Caught in the tangled web of depression, he must have felt there was nothing to look forward to, no promise of change. And so young.

I had read about depression and suicide in medical school, but until now I had not encountered either at first hand. It was a puzzling and humbling experience. The stark reality of such despair in a world where so much seemed possible would continue to haunt me, and it motivated me to try to better understand the mysteries of the human mind.

Such dark and morbid thoughts had no place in my upbringing. I had spent my early years in Trondheim, a city of forty thousand—Norway's third-largest. Trondheim still has a patrician air, with its wide streets, old trees and low houses. I loved its austere beauty; I loved the building in which I attended school, an eight-hundred-year-old structure whose walls were several feet thick; I loved the nearby cathedral, begun in the eleventh century. Tradition and stability surrounded me.

Although I came from a family of eleven children, I never felt I lacked for attention. Indeed, as the firstborn I even suspected I might be my mother's favorite.

For the most part, my childhood was busy, secure and happy, if uneventful.

When I was eight I came down with pneumonia, which kept me in bed for weeks. Over and over I was told, "You'll get well, but it will take time." I was miserable away from my school and classmates. In that era before antibiotics, the strong-tasting medicine that was poured down my throat periodically along with quantities of aspirin seemed to do little to hasten the day I could resume a normal life.

Weeks of convalescence turned into months before I regained my health. But the mystery of illness stayed with me. Why had I been sick so long? Why wasn't there a cure for pneumonia? My curiosity was piqued.

Another incident was less dramatic, but just as important. It was my first trip to the library. It is significant that of all the books I could have chosen to read, the one I picked was about Stanley and Livingstone in Africa, a story of a quest, against great odds, to track down someone who was thought to be inaccessible. Stanley was a kind of detective: that intrigued and excited me. That story, in fact, was a model for what I would be doing later when, as a physician, I would need to discover the hidden identity and cause of sickness; and later still when, working as a psychiatrist, I would have to track down the inaccessible person of the unconscious.

When I was ten, my budding scientific curiosity got some encouragement—and direction—from a very wise

17

teacher. We were on a train for a class outing, and as usual, I had my nose buried in a book, oblivious to the beautiful countryside. He pulled me away from my absorption with the printed word and gently reminded me that nature was also out there to be "read."

By age thirteen I had made my decision, and one day after school I breathlessly announced to my father that I wanted to be a doctor.

He greeted my declaration with respect. "That is a noble profession," he said, but added, "I thought you'd become a banker."

I was horrified. "A *banker*?" I exclaimed. "But I don't know anything about money." In truth, I didn't know much about doctors either.

As I moved into adolescence, the sunny glow that had surrounded my youth became tempered by the realization that there was another side of life. I immersed myself in the study of this darkness, in Ibsen's and Strindberg's plays and the anguished art of Edvard Munch. Hidden motivation and underlying complexity, contrast, contradiction and ambivalence took on a fascination for me that I retain to this day.

I discovered the Danish philosopher Sören Kierkegaard, whose religious and moralistic musings did not interest me so much as his insight into the darker side of the human mind. And Dostoevsky, in *Crime and Punishment*—how had he created this killer who sought so eagerly to be punished? Had the author read his own mind? Dostoevsky did me a great service, opening my eyes to the world of anger, conspiracy, hatred and duplicity, murder and guilt. It was the inner world of man, a mental underworld, the familiar province of the criminal mind that was to become the focus of much of my life's work.

I spent seven years at the Royal Frederick University (now the University of Oslo). Increasingly I discovered vast areas of my own ignorance as I struggled to master my studies; but at the same time I was becoming aware of my strengths, one of which would be particularly useful as my work branched into psychiatry. It was at this time that I began to develop a very sharp intuitive faculty. For a doctor it is a godsend, that sixth sense so desperately needed in the effort to diagnose a difficult case. And for a forensic psychiatrist, it's the knack for smelling a rat.

Intuition, of course, is not enough. Thorough examination and research are always necessary. But that ability to get an early sense of what is going on with a person or a case can provide a real head start.

Only recently, for example, intuition helped me in a case in which a lawyer's tax evasion had been attributed to epilepsy. I sensed something not quite right when I first met him, but I couldn't immediately put my finger on it. Then I realized that he appeared to be hardly breathing as he spoke—four or five breaths a minute, when the normal rhythm was fifteen or sixteen. I took his blood pressure and found it to be critically high. The constant sleepiness he complained of was due to impairment of the oxygen supply to his brain. I suspected that he had sleep apnea syndrome, not epilepsy, and that his inability to concentrate, caused by the disease, was ruining his law practice as well as preventing him from dealing with his taxes. Because something about him had seemed to be unusual, I had done a physical examination that ordinarily I might not have, and my diagnosis was confirmed at a sleep-disorder clinic. Consequently, instead of going to prison the man underwent treatment for his sleep problem.

II

After graduation, I was eager to test my intuitive abilities in psychiatric practice, then a relatively new field. But at that time a young doctor in Norway could not pursue any specialized studies until he had been in general practice for a year or had served as a public-health doctor. I did both.

For a newly minted physician, the world is full of curious cases—he is seeing everything for the first time. Even so, I dealt in those early years with a few that were pretty strange.

One of my first patients couldn't tell me what was wrong with her—she was very young, about sixteen, and in great pain, but couldn't speak. She lay on her bed in a small farmhouse in the country. Her mouth was half open, and she was trying to speak, but I couldn't understand her. It was obvious that she couldn't move her jaw.

There was no precedent in my meager experience for such a situation. By the dim light of a small kerosene lamp I began to examine the girl. I put my fingers in her mouth, remembering that we had been taught to be careful in this procedure not to extend our fingers past the teeth; otherwise, a sudden closing of the jaw could result in disaster.

It occurred to me that her jaw might be out of joint, and so I tried manipulating it. Suddenly it snapped shut, almost catching my fingers. In my diagnosis, treatment and narrow escape, I had been the beneficiary of beginner's luck.

At once my patient began to talk, as though she couldn't stop.

"I was so bored," she said. "Today was Saturday and I had a date tonight, but my father wouldn't let me go out, so I had to stay home. I yawned and yawned, and then all of a sudden my mouth wouldn't go back together."

That didn't leave me much room for medical advice, but I suggested she restrain her yawning in the future.

Other cases were more grave. A woman of about fifty came to see me about a sore on her breast. My examination revealed a tumorlike bulge beneath it. It's a cancer, I thought. I told her I couldn't treat it, and said that she must go as soon as possible to the hospital in Trondheim. She protested, but I pleaded with her, warning that she could be in great danger, and she finally relented. A few days later, the woman's sister came to see me—with an identical growth in her breast. This time I did not have to plead with her to enter the hospital. Sadly, it was too late for both.

In those valleys and mountains, I saw more than my share of incurable diseases and the constant struggle of life against death. Sometimes entire villages were depopulated—their inhabitants along with their livestock dying en masse of tuberculosis.

When I finally became a psychiatrist and opened an office in Oslo, I at least had a general grounding in medical practice. And while I had learned over and over again that things were rarely as simple as they appeared on the surface, I was to discover that often the best way to work with the labyrinth of the human mind is to reduce a problem to a series of simple elements, then deal with each in turn. As I gained experience as a psychiatrist, I also learned that often the most powerful weapon for healing was the element of surprise.

One of my patients, a married, middle-aged, almost destitute Jewish refugee from Nazi oppression in Germany, was severely depressed. He saw no future for himself, had no hope. Given his circumstances, that was understandable, although he did have prospects of emigrating to the United States.

Through psychotherapy, and with the aid of medication, I was able to lift his depression somewhat, but he was still unable to sleep. He had lost a considerable amount of weight, and his health had deteriorated so badly that he viewed his trip to the United States as a potential threat to his life. He denied having suicidal thoughts, but in one of his biweekly therapy sessions he seemed to be edging toward that state, weeping and despairing of his existence. Consolation wouldn't do.

Walking slowly to the door, he turned and looked at me. "I will kill myself," he said.

"It's too late," I declared.

"It *is*?" he inquired, taken aback.

"Yes."

Visibly shaken, he left my office without another word. In truth, I didn't know what he might do, and I feared for his life. But as it happened, he seemed to accept the pronouncement that it was too late for suicide as a promise of sorts that he might still attain some peace in his life. Perhaps he reasoned that if his life had moved beyond the point of suicide, then he must have a future, with a chance to restore his self-esteem. Sometimes the healing process begins with the simplest remark or thought.

Often it was hard to believe that such a simple, straightforward approach could be so effective for people with complex problems. But it was, over and over again. A twenty-five-year-old girl who had been depressed and unhappy for some time came to see me. As a preliminary to therapy, I advised her to go to the country for a restful vacation. A few days later she called me at two o'clock in the morning.

"Everything is so hopeless," her weak voice came faintly over the wire. "I'm going to kill myself." There was a long pause, and then she said, "I'm going to drown myself."

"No, you can't do that," I told her. "The water is too cold."

"Cold?" she repeated, uncertainly.

"Yes, very cold," I said. "Why don't you take the train tomorrow morning, and my nurse and I will be waiting for you at the station to take you to the hospital."

"You think so, Doctor?" she asked. Her voice now held a quaver of hope.

She did meet us at the station. She was glad to see us and was shortly thereafter admitted to a hospital. What she had really needed and unconsciously wanted was assurance that someone cared enough to want to help her. By telling her that I didn't want her to go into the water because it was too cold—an absurd bit of reasoning under the circumstances—I had shown her that I was interested in her welfare. Once she was safely in the hospital, we could proceed with more conventional therapy.

Some of my cases would have been almost comical if they had not been tragic. A woman had been referred to me because she had a stiff finger, and the referring physician begged me to see her that day. What a strange reason, I thought, for a psychiatric referral.

23

The woman who came to my office was attractive and well dressed. She sat down opposite me and immediately placed her right hand on my desk with her index finger pointing straight into the air. In an effort to hide my surprise, I began to ask about her family. Did she have children?

"Two," she answered, but added nothing about their sex or ages. I sensed that she was holding in a great deal of resentment and anger, and I thought that this preliminary examination would not be very fruitful. Nevertheless, appearing as if I hadn't noticed either her stiff finger or her hostility, I continued with the interview for nearly an hour, while she sat before me, stiff and unbending—both her finger and her attitude.

I asked about her relationship with her husband. She said that everything was all right with her marriage.

"Why do you think you have a stiff finger?" I inquired.

No answer. Then I asked about her grandparents, aunts, uncles and her relationship with her parents. By now nearly two hours had gone by, while she continued to sit quietly, finger in the air, responding to my questions as briefly as possible.

Finally, I asked: "Can you show me how the finger looked before it became stiff?"

"Oh," she answered, with some animation, "it was this way." And she curled it easily into her palm.

For a second, she stared at her finger in surprise. But in the next instant, realizing what she had done, she was overwhelmed by anger and indignation. She bolted from the chair and ran from the office. I had forced her to see that her finger didn't have to be stiff. She had experienced a temporary release from the compulsion that had kept it pointing straight up in the air.

To me it was perfectly clear (as it would be later to her) that she was suffering from a deep-seated neurosis, but the first step toward therapy had been taken; healing had begun. Once again I had been reminded that in the art of healing, very few things were to be taken for granted. Each patient was a unique mystery, whose plot had to be carefully unraveled.

During these early years, I was becoming aware of how much more there was to learn about the human psyche. In the mid-1930s I spent some time at the Tavistock Clinic in London, and while I was there I studied anthropology with Bronislav Malinowski, one of the pioneers in the field. Malinowski's lectures were enlightening, but in his unwillingness to acknowledge the role of the sexual drive in human behavior, he seemed to me to miss a crucial element in the configuration of personality.

I would have gone to Vienna for psychoanalytical training with Freud, but the rapid ascendancy of Hitler and Nazism made travel for me, as a Jew, very dangerous.

Although I could not see Freud personally, he was gracious enough to correspond with me about cases in which we shared an interest.

It would not be long before I would need all my wits and energy to preserve my own and my family's safety— from Hitler. But for the time being, I was immersed in my new love, psychiatry.

In 1938 I was presented with a splendid opportunity to further that interest. I was engaged by Dr. Johan Scharffenberg, the chief psychiatrist in the Department of Justice at Oslo, to assist him in his research into criminal behavior. An outspoken foe of communism, Nazism, capitalism and every other "ism," he spoke out against injustice wherever he encountered it. Well informed in his own field, and highly literate in others as well, Scharffenberg also impressed me with his phenomenal memory. I was fascinated by our research into criminal behavior. Criminals were baffling, enigmatic and, at least initially, unpredictable.

Norway in the 1930s had a homogeneous population of only 2.5 million. Criminals were rare and crimes were infrequent. The country's criminal laws stressed rehabilitation rather than punishment; there was no death penalty, and prison sentences were mild. Still, we had our share of burglars, robbers and rapists; and once in a while we saw a counterfeiter, arsonist or murderer.

In one case, a seemingly normal, quiet forty-two-year-old man had murdered his wife with an ax, in an unpredictable eruption of bloody rage.

He was his wife's intellectual inferior; they had married because she had become pregnant. A factory worker, he brought home only a modest paycheck; she had never been satisfied with the amount of money he gave her and had nagged him constantly. She had objected to his visits to his parents and scolded him for it, but she had felt no compunction about leaving him with their four children and going off to visit her family.

Her out-of-work relatives had begun to use their home as a hotel. First one of her sisters had stayed with them for a long time; then another—with three children—had taken up residence. The house always seemed overcrowded, and life at home had swiftly degenerated into not much more than a war of nerves. He seemed to take his onslaught calmly, however, and showed no resentment.

At that point, two things happened which may have

tipped the balance. He was led to believe that his wife was carrying on an affair with another man. At the same time, the state of their finances dictated that he take on a second job. Finally, he was at the end of his tether emotionally and physically. One day, when his wife was nagging him about his inability to support his family, he calmly gave her the money she asked for. Then he hacked her to death with the ax.

The judge in the case, recognizing extenuating circumstances, gave him a light sentence. The murderer, the court contended, had acted not so much out of criminal will as from harassment and mental torture.

The truth, it seemed to me, was a bit more complex. It was true that he had been pushed far past the breaking point. On the other hand, if things were so horrible, he could have left his wife before he reached that point. He could have borne some responsibility for his own life. But instead of meeting his problems head on, he had resorted to a kind of passive masochistic withdrawal. Finally, his marital situation had produced such a volatile brew that the inevitable explosion had occurred. Although I could sympathize with his suffering, I felt that he might have been held more responsible for his part in the tragedy.

Occasionally we read of the murder of an unwanted infant. In this case the child was the result of an affair between a fifty-year-old man and the housemaid who worked on his farm. After she gave birth he strangled the infant, hid its body under the bed that night and buried it the following day behind the barn.

The murderer was a dwarf. He stood three feet, two inches high. Although his torso was normally developed, his arms and legs were abnormally short. As a youngster he had been a loner, largely withdrawn into his own world, and had daydreamed excessively. He grew up obsessed with unfulfilled wishes and hopes, and matured into a man possessed of an overwhelming degree of self-loathing. Afraid that the infant would have his own deformity, he killed it. The court, taking the entire situation into account, chose to be lenient.

Crimes rooted in passion or mental defect were not the only kinds of cases we handled; there were also offenders whose mental state was a product of their criminal nature, malingerers who faked insanity to avoid prison. In one such case, a paradigm for many that I would handle later, a tall, good-looking, calculating and seductive man had thoroughly convinced doctors and judges that he was sick. He made a profession out of promising marriage to rich women, from whom he would steal as much as he could before leaving town. When not headed for the altar, he spent a great deal of time in mental hospitals being "cured." He was in jail following his latest amorous adventure when we encountered him; specifically, he was in an isolation cell because he had been carrying on like a lunatic. An unwanted child, he was genuinely antisocial in his behavior; but he had no authentic hallucinations or delusions, and from our examination of him we concluded that he knew what he was doing. His was a case more of acting than of acting out, and as a result of our findings he was sent to prison.

My work with Scharffenberg provided me with valuable exposure to the criminal mind. Unfortunately, in those troubled times one encountered the underside of human nature just by opening a newspaper or listening to the radio. The Nazi shadow over Europe was growing longer.

When the Germans invaded Norway on April 9, 1940, I found myself in a personal struggle of life and death.

A journalist friend, hearing the news of the attack, called and warned me to get out of the country. My wife, Lova, and I, however, wanted to stay and fight Hitler. We took our two daughters, Inger and Annemarie, aged seven and three, and headed north toward the mountains. We worked with the Army to set up a field hospital. I did my best to treat casualties with the equipment available to me, and Lova worked as cook, ambulance driver, nurse—whatever was needed.

The resistance was brave, but inevitably futile. The news was consistently bad; and we knew at last that we would have to leave Norway for America, while there was still time. Our leavetaking was not without its share of fear and personal loss, but with the help of dear friends and wonderful strangers, and a little luck too, we were able to make our way to what would be our new home.

III

I arrived in New York hopeful and determined to succeed; but the only thing certain about my professional career at this point was uncertainty. With the help of friends, I secured a job in Chicago at the psychiatric diagnostic section of the Joliet State Penitentiary, for which I qualified without an examination, and our family made its way to our new home in the Midwest. My job was to diagnose and submit a full report on all new prisoners, six or seven each day. Not an easy task, and time constraints made it even harder: I had to be out of the building by three-thirty, when the prisoners were locked up.

One of the first things I inquired about when I began working at Joliet was the kind of prisoners held by the state. "All kinds," a guard informed me: "murderers, robbers, embezzlers, rapists—the worst kind." "Any particular ones of interest?" I asked. "Well, there's Nathan Leopold," he replied. Leopold was then housed at Statesville Prison in Joliet. The Leopold and Loeb thrill-killing—"the crime of the century" it had been called in the innocent days of the 1920s—had been big news in Norway. I was fascinated by Leopold's proximity and the possibility that I might have access to him. Little did I know that I would eventually play an important role in his life—a life which had so far been a tragic waste.

The working conditions at Joliet were less than ideal, and after a year we decided that we would be better situated in New York, where Professor Nolan D. C. Lewis of the Psychiatric Institute at Columbia University asked me to give postgraduate courses. I accepted, and began to work toward my New York State certification. I also spent some months in Topeka, Kansas, at the Menninger Clinic while on a one-year leave of absence from Columbia.

But my career was in New York. Clearly the center of American psychiatry, and because of its famous clinics, hospitals and other institutions and its large, dense population, New York offered the best opportunity to practice forensic psychiatry, a field about to come into its own. Where better to study the wide spectrum of human behavior than at the world-famous Bellevue Hospital? The director of its psychiatric department offered me a job, and I gladly accepted it. Every night, between the hours of midnight and 8 A.M., a wave of the emotionally disturbed and often violent elements of the population passed through that institution. Schizophrenia, alcoholism, suicide, drug abuse and murder—they were as routine at Bellevue as the common cold is in the office of a general practitioner. I saw fifteen to thirty people a night, each case with its unique elements of tragedy and despair, and most with very little hope.

Before long I was transferred to the psychiatric clinic of the Court of General Sessions, where my work reminded me of my stint at Joliet. From nine until two each day I examined five to seven offenders and gave the judge a presentencing report on each. It was hard work and usually, of necessity, too superficial. Clarifying the mental state of any individual takes time, and even more so when he has no desire to cooperate. But the job was advantageous in that I could apply what I had learned of human pathology to difficult cases and begin to hone my diagnostic skills in the science of forensic psychiatry.

Occasionally, when a case was considered difficult and important enough, the examining psychiatrist was allowed more time to interview the convicted man or woman. Such was the case when I confronted Wayne Lonergan, a tall, handsome, well-groomed (his fingers were always manicured) and muscular playboy with a broad but somewhat phony smile, whose conviction of second-degree homicide in killing his beautiful and socially prominent wife had been front-page news. Lonergan was to be the second murderer I had dealt with who had achieved widespread notoriety.

Typically, at this time, a psychiatrist making a presentencing report concentrated less on formulating an entire picture of a person's motives and character than on

31

simply classifying him on the broad spectrum from normal to psychotic. But I thought the portrait needed to be fleshed out. Simple diagnostic labels were necessary to satisfy the law, but they would not always tell a judge the full story. More than that, I felt that too much reliance on classification could also encourage a certain laxity in the examination. Habitual criminals are often artful manipulators, and many a psychiatrist has been outfoxed by a knowledgeable and clever offender.

In addition to interviewing the prisoner, I felt it was necessary to question his friends and relatives and to delve as thoroughly as possible into his background, through whatever research was relevant. It was the psychiatrist's counterpart of the work the detectives had done originally to crack the case. In fact, the psychiatrist becomes a kind of detective, tracking down not the culprit, who is already in custody, but the source of the criminal's actions. As this more rigorous approach was observed by others, more and more psychiatrists incorporated it into the emerging profession of forensic psychiatry.

When I applied these methods to Wayne Lonergan, I came up with a portrait of a man whose good looks were truly only skin-deep. The inner man was ugly, exploitative and totally amoral.

He denied killing his wife. Not that he hadn't wished for her death: it was no secret that they did not get along. He claimed he had been at a concert when the murder occurred; as proof, he even produced some ticket stubs. But the police later established that he had left the concert before it was over. He claimed that he had then picked up a soldier on the street and spent the night with him. This proved to be a lie. When he returned home, his wife informed him that she was cutting off his allowance, his sole means of support. In the wild argument that followed, Lonergan hit her on the head with a candelabrum. Dr. Milton Helpern stated at the trial that death was caused by asphyxia by strangulation, laceration of the scalp, fracture of the skull, and bruises of the brain.

The argument had begun over money, grown heated, gone out of control and ended in murder—a fairly common and simple crime. But it was not so simple, and there was a good deal more than money involved.

By delving into Lonergan's past I was able to piece together the bizarre story of his life. He had come to New York from his native Canada. He hesitated when I asked him how he had supported himself, but finally described the life of a gigolo and prostitute, who earned his keep through sexual activity with anyone willing to pay the price.

Lonergan took on all comers—men, women, even transvestites who received him in feminine boudoirs, perfumed and adorned with ankle bracelets and earrings. His eyes glittered with excitement when he described the women who had pursued him. They were fascinated by his sexuality and even after his conviction for murder wrote passionate letters to him.

Lonergan had a dual style with women. He was cool and aloof, playing hard to get; but at the same time he managed to convey a helplessness which almost always elicited a mothering response from his women. There was, apparently, something very appealing about this helpless little boy.

The real little boy in him had been deprived as well as helpless; getting what he had not been given in childhood

33

was the central motivation of Lonergan's adult life. His father had been a weak man who had very little to do with his son. The boy had become dependent on his mother; but she was as self-centered as her son grew up to be, and offered him little but rejection. Thus Lonergan felt impelled to constantly seek from others the attention he never got at home. At the same time, he had few resources of his own other than the facile charm he used to manipulate people.

He was himself incapable of offering affection to anyone. His only expression of genuine emotion occurred in our last interview, when he cried at the mention of his mother, whom he felt he had disgraced.

In my report to the court I described him as an antisocial man with a character disorder. His wife had known of his active "social" life, which had continued after their marriage, and they had quarreled bitterly over his behavior. The quarrel over money had been only the last straw. But had she known of his strangest relationship? Of that I could never be sure.

Gradually in my interviews with him, Lonergan began to hint that the circumstances under which he had met his future wife were peculiar, to say the least. He had been working in Atlantic City, pushing carts along the boardwalk. In the course of this job he had cultivated the friendship of a wealthy vacationing brewer who had achieved international notoriety with his Paris parties. Soon after meeting him, Lonergan quit his job and went to live with this patron. The press was abuzz with scandalous rumors of a sexual relationship between the two men, and according to one account from the New York *Journal American* of February 20, 1944:

Lonergan now numbered dozens of wealthy, bored play-
boys and madcap girls among his friends in this subnormal
life....His satisfaction vanished and was replaced with
higher ambitions when he first met Patricia Burton, the
spoiled daughter of Bill Burton. Burton was alarmed by
Lonergan's attentions to his daughter. He threatened to end
his patronage. He argued in vain with Patricia.

Laughingly the debutante once told her friends in a
nightclub: "I am going to marry Wayne. If he's good enough
for my father, he's good enough for me." In the winter of
1941 Burton died and the road to marriage was opened to
Lonergan.

She was the woman Lonergan married and murdered.

In our last interview, Lonergan, a cigarette dangling
from his mouth, asked my opinion as to the length of the
sentence he was likely to get. While I wasn't sure, I guessed
that the judge might hand down thirty-five years for his
conviction for second-degree homicide. He let out a su-
perior laugh. "I won't get more than seven," he told me
confidently. The next day, sentence was passed: thirty-
five years. Several years later, when I was doing research
on sex offenders at Sing Sing Prison, I saw Lonergan. He
had little to say and seemed resigned to his fate.

The length of the sentence did not surprise me. I had
learned how a judge took into account the specific nature
of the person and the crime in meting out justice. Lonergan's offense was not one motivated by momentary passion or anger; and his personality did not suggest the
likelihood of fairly quick rehabilitation. But I *was* dis-
mayed that neither the prosecution nor the defense had
ever touched on aspects of his family life at his trial—as
if that were irrelevant to passing judgment.

Such subjects should be central to the judicial process, I thought. But human development in the formative years and its ultimate relationship to criminal behavior were still virtually unknown territory.

During these years, forensic psychiatrists had to break much new ground. First we had to make decisions about the defendant's state of mind: was he madman or malingerer? But even when the veracity of a person could be reasonably determined, what about his motivation? If the person was insane, what had made him that way? If he was feigning insanity, what was his real motivation?

After the Lonergan case, I was frequently asked to consult in cases where an offender's motivation and state of mind were hard to determine. I was gratified by the acceptance our relatively new profession was gaining.

In focusing on the family as a fundamental influence on children, I was unconsciously drawing on the circumstances of my own life. A whole galaxy of cousins, aunts and uncles had surrounded my large immediate family. Even as a child, I had been acutely aware of how we all influenced each other. I was confident that careful study would demonstrate similar influences, even in situations less benign than mine had been.

In 1944 I began a project with the Psychiatric Institute of Columbia University to study the influence of family on neurotic, psychotic and criminal behavior. We believed the family to be a fundamental influence on children, and our project involved the study of about a hundred juvenile delinquents and their families, along with a control group of equal size consisting of nonoffenders. The work involved was enormous—we worked long hours, and nights and weekends were spoken for. My memory of that time, however, is one of exhilaration rather than exhaustion. No one had ever studied both offenders and their families. We were pioneers.

In the course of the study we employed every technique that seemed relevant: standard psychological tests, such as the Rorschach (ink-blot interpretation) test, physical examinations and extensive psychological interviews. Slowly, the patterns became clear. Among the delinquents and their families, we discovered that one or another troubling situation (and often many of them in combination) could be expected: one parent dominated the family, often to the point of physical abuse; a parent drank; one child was preferred over another; still another child hadn't been wanted at all—our findings were depressingly consistent. Frequently, both the children and their parents in the first group exhibited marked feelings of hatred, fear, revenge, rejection and abandonment. Jealousy and hostility between members of a problem family were common. While some of these conditions were also to be found in the control group, they were never present to the degree that they were in the families with delinquent children.

The conclusions of the Columbia University Forum for the Study of Juvenile Delinquency and Crime, as the project was formally known, were published in 1949. Family tension or disturbance, it was clear to us, was the basic cause of juvenile delinquency and criminal behavior. Effective treatment to undo the neurosis or psychosis caused by that conflict required treatment of the families as a whole, and not just their younger and more overtly wayward members. Our findings produced far-ranging repercussions among sociologists, psychologists and psychiatrists. The years of hard work had certainly been worthwhile.

I continued to be very busy in my private practice and

in my public career as a forensic psychiatrist. And I found myself testifying just as often as a witness for the prosecution as for the defense. I was very much aware how the term "insanity" might be used—and abused—in the courtroom. Too often criminals who have been labeled "insane" seem to "get away with murder." For many of us, the term is associated with "walking off scot-free." It is true that there is a whole breed of lawbreakers who prey on society's willingness to look for extenuating circumstances in the commission of a crime by someone with an aberrant mental state. But it is just as true that some people really cannot be responsible for their actions under certain circumstances.

A good part of my career has been devoted to making these determinations in criminal cases. I have studied both extremes and all the murky areas in between; I have spent hundreds of hours in courtrooms and prisons with genuinely troubled individuals, and with others who were just waiting to take advantage of any loophole in the law they could find. And although I've worked with notorious criminals whose exploits made front-page headlines, I've found much to learn and marvel at in my experiences with the more anonymous.

My personal life had taken on a serenity and everyday quality that I welcomed. But my career as a forensic psychiatrist began to produce a kind of creative turmoil that I also embraced. As I became more involved with prominent cases, I found myself embroiled in the issues and debates that swirled around the controversial topic of criminal insanity. The cases on which I worked addressed very directly the concept of responsibility. The lessons they taught—and the sometimes bizarre characteristics of the human mind they revealed—are part of the debate that rages to this day over what to do when a crime may have been committed out of something other than criminal intent.

2
THE LEOPOLD-LOEB MURDER CASE

On the afternoon of May 21, 1924, in Chicago, Nathan Leopold, whose future seemed full of promise, and his friend and lover, Richard Loeb, both eighteen years old, kidnapped fourteen-year-old Bobby Franks, and Loeb beat him to death. They stripped the body from the waist down, and although the evidence is inconclusive, one or both of them probably performed a sexual act on it. Several hours later they buried Bobby Franks in a cistern under a railway track.

In the perspective of all that has happened since the 1920s, the murder of Bobby Franks hardly qualifies as the crime of the century, as it was seen then. But at that time the brutality and senselessness of the act exploded like a bomb in the public consciousness. People began to realize that society was changing in some frightening way. The youth of the two murderers (this was the beginning of the tidal wave that came to be called juvenile delinquency), the sexual undercurrent of their crime and the fact that theirs was the first major trial to use the testimony of psychiatrists on the background and state of mind of a defendant made an indelible impression on the millions who followed the sensational case in the newspapers.

The first time I met Nathan Leopold—at Statesville Prison in Illinois in 1941—it was out of curiosity. I was a young psychiatrist at the beginning of a career that would bring me constantly into contact with the criminal mind; he was one of the most notorious criminals of his time, with a mind whose breadth and power had often been remarked on. He had been a brilliant boy. At the age of ten he had already written a booklet on birds; at sixteen he had entered the University of Michigan, where he studied psychology, Russian, French, Greek, Latin, Spanish, German and Sanskrit. He could speak knowledgeably on a wide range of subjects—politics, the Depression, the law, jazz. As an adult he was to correspond with many people, including university professors who wished to discuss their specialties with him.

If a prison could be thought of as beautiful, then the institution that held Nathan Leopold qualified. The large white structure resembled a splendid hotel, an impression that its marble-faced main hall did not dispel, although the effect was certainly tempered by the bars and the numerous guards.

I had expected Leopold to be taller than his five feet, six inches. He was slender, with observant eyes set in a smallish face. In our first conversation (there were to be several), we touched on a wide range of topics—everything, that is, but the reason for his having spent the past seventeen years in prison: obviously the one thing I wanted most to know about. He was as intelligent and well read as I had imagined. He spoke freely, seemed to be in an expansive mood and appeared to be at peace with himself. If anything, prison seemed to agree with him.

When I tried to get him to address the circumstances surrounding the crime, he let me know, courteously but firmly, that he did not intend to talk about his past. I didn't press the point, but I did tell him that my interest in the case dated from the time I had first read the newspaper accounts in Norway. He was a bit startled that the facts had been reported in such detail in a place that far from Chicago.

Then I sought to discuss his lover, Richard Loeb, who had been slashed to death in prison in 1936. Again Leopold fended me off. He stared at me intently, as if trying to analyze my motivation. Finally, he did allow that he was aware that his case might have been the first in which a complete psychological investigation of offenders had been undertaken, and he obviously understood the reason for my intense interest.

And that was about all I could get out of him in the way of substance until, more than a decade later, I came to play a direct role in what was left of his life.

In the intervening years he was often on my mind. I studied contemporary accounts of the crime and the trial, particularly the interviews and examinations made by an eminent psychiatrist, Dr. William Alanson White, superintendent of St. Elizabeth's Hospital in Washington, D.C. And I thought a good deal about my own brief encounter with one of the most curious figures in the history of American crime.

II

The Leopolds lived on Chicago's then fashionable South Side in a large, impressive house. The father was a well-to-do, respectable businessman—although there were a few broken branches on his side of the family tree: two relatives were psychotic. His interaction with his son does not appear to have played a big role in the boy's development, but all evidence points to a very difficult and significant relationship between Nathan and his mother. He seems to have been a demanding child, precocious and egocentric, enthralled with his sense of his own importance, ready to exploit her, assuming that she would do his bidding.

Nathan's mother died when he was five years old—a loss from which he never fully recovered. In his grief, according to Dr. White's findings, he began to idealize and worship her. He also felt considerable remorse for the way that he had treated her. The more he idealized his mother, the guiltier he felt; she was on a pedestal, he a base and lowly person. Her passing locked him into infantile feelings of psychological dependence; instead of freeing himself from the normally close attachment of early childhood, he became bound to her.

The governess who took over his upbringing did not help him break those ties; he treated her as he had his mother. The young Jewish boy was very much taken with her devout Catholicism, especially her veneration of the Virgin Mary. He adopted her worship of Mary and infused it with feelings that were actually directed at the memory of his mother. His ideal woman—distant, unattainable

44

and perfect—was a fantasy that prevented him from developing a genuine interest in real women as he grew older.

Although he told the psychiatrists who examined him that he had had many girlfriends, it seemed unlikely that he had ever in fact had a true love affair.

Later, in his memoirs, *Life Plus 99 Years*, Leopold wrote of a romantic encounter the day before his arrest:

> We had dinner at a wayside inn, Connie and I. By now I knew her favorite dishes, and I felt about ten feet tall talking over the details of ordering. She smiled appreciatively, tenderly. And then we rented a canoe and went out on the Des Plaines River. I had brought my ukulele, and Connie accompanied herself as she sang softly to me. She had a lovely voice. But then everything about her was lovely.
>
> We found the perfect nook, a grassy glen surrounded by thick woods. Here we beached the canoe. Connie had brought the blue vellum-covered volume of French poetry I had given her for her birthday the week before. And as she read the liquid verses to me, I laid my head in her lap. Lamartine has never had a lovelier interpreter.
>
> Perhaps the weather was perfect, maybe the sun was shining softly. I could see only those luminous, twilight-shadowed brown eyes, could hear only those limpid French verses uttered in that mellifluous voice.

This passage sounds lovely, idyllic—too idyllic to be true. Leopold may have *wanted* to be in love with her; maybe he had even tried to talk himself into it—but he was simply not capable of sustaining such a relationship at this point in his life.

His friend Richard Loeb had similar problems. He too was highly intelligent, came from a wealthy family and had a second cousin who had been committed to a mental institution. Richard's paternal grandfather had beaten his children severely, possibly accounting for the fact that Richard's father was very lenient with his children. Richard had also been raised by a governess, a strict woman with whom he developed an intense bond, according to psychiatrists who later examined him. He identified with her, and it was a jolting experience for him when, in his nineteenth year, she left.

For Loeb, however, signs warning of a troubled adulthood were everywhere apparent. His youth was filled with episodes of thievery: he began by stealing small sums of money at home, branched out to shoplifting, worked up to stealing liquor from friends of the family, then graduated to car theft. From there, it wasn't too far to arson. He was never caught at any of this, which encouraged him to pursue his budding criminal career.

Loeb envisioned himself as a supremely intelligent person who could perform great deeds. His ambition was nothing less than to be the greatest criminal of the twentieth century. But as with many people whose fantasies run to the grandiose, he paid the price with great anxiety and insecurity. He had strong, unresolved feelings of guilt and a deep-seated, unconscious wish to be punished for his wrongdoing. Even as a child he had recurring morbid fantasies of being confined in a jail. And as with Leopold, the masculine, potent front he presented to the world was paper-thin.

Leopold and Loeb became friends at the University of Michigan. They seemed almost fated to meet. Their family backgrounds and emotional makeup were similar, and their sexual fantasies played into each other's needs. They were, perhaps, fatally attracted, and when they met they fell in love.

Their attachment was passionate and deep. Leopold, who felt he could not live without his friend, transferred the fantasized relationship with his mother to Loeb. As he had idealized his mother and sought to grovel at her feet, so he attached himself to his lover, seeking only to play the slave to Loeb's king. Loeb the stronger, Leopold the weaker—they fitted like key and lock.

Leopold worshiped Loeb's intelligence, too. He abdicated his own need to think and accepted almost anything his mentor suggested—social or antisocial, innocent or criminal. From the beginning, they were partners in crime. They fell out on only one notable occasion. In November 1923, they burglarized Loeb's fraternity house on the campus of the University of Michigan in Ann Arbor. Somehow this crime left them very much unsatisfied, and they began to quarrel, even threatening each other with a separation. For one of the few times in their relationship, Leopold felt rebellious.

For Leopold, the only satisfactory resolution of their conflict was to be found in strengthening Loeb's domination. Now it was to be complete, and whenever Loeb used the code phrase "for Richard's sake," Leopold was to yield.

Loeb's needs were harder to define. The petty crimes brought less and less satisfaction, and he was becoming increasingly depressed, even toying with the notion of committing suicide. They decided to up the ante.

Kidnapping was the next step. They mulled it over for

a while, and contemplated seizing Loeb's father or younger brother, but they abandoned that idea as being too difficult to bring off.

Shortly afterward, however, they came close to putting their general plan into effect. They rented a car and drove around Chicago, looking for a possible victim. At one point they actually picked up a little boy, but apparently did not find him interesting enough and let him go. Finally, they settled on a boy who lived nearby. "Bob" was president of his school class, thus making him a worthier target than just any stranger. Fortunately for him, he was in school when the duo set out to get him.

The first Bob being out of reach, they settled on another. Bobby Franks, the son of a millionaire who lived in the same neighborhood as Leopold and Loeb, would be their victim.

The crime that shocked the world was over rather quickly. At about five o'clock on the afternoon of May 14, with Leopold driving, Loeb grabbed young Franks off the street, pushed him into the backseat of the car, impulsively hit him over the head—although violence had not been part of their plan—and killed him.

After the body was buried, they followed through on their scheme. Both of them crowded into a phone booth, and Leopold dialed Bobby Franks's home; calling himself "Frank Johnson," he told the anxious parents that their son had been kidnapped. A letter would follow in the morning, he said, with instructions about the ransom. They had already prepared the letter, which demanded ten thousand dollars, and now they sent it off, special delivery.

The next day, when they met for lunch, Loeb was in

high spirits. The Bobby Franks kidnapping was front-page news. Leopold, in his memoirs, described his partner as "exuberant. All keyed up." They thought they had committed the perfect crime. "Let's see them unravel this one," Loeb exulted.

Within a few days, however, everything had indeed unraveled, and their carefully constructed fantasy of the perfect crime collapsed in ruins. The police had found a pair of horn-rimmed glasses near the remote spot where the body was discovered. At first they were thought to be Bobby Franks's, but when that proved not to be the case, the police theorized, correctly, that they belonged to the murderer.

It was a fluke, Leopold wrote later in his book. Ordinarily he didn't wear glasses, but six months earlier, plagued by recurring headaches and believing they were the result of eyestrain from his studies, he had obtained a pair for reading. He had worn them for only three or four weeks, until the headaches ceased. He thought he had left them in an old jacket, but in fact they had been in the topcoat he had worn on the day of the crime. He had dropped the coat, Loeb had picked it up and in the process the glasses had fallen from the pocket.

Still, they both thought, it would be impossible to trace the ownership of the glasses—"one in a jillion," as Leopold put it in his memoirs. Nevertheless, they were traced, and through an incredible coincidence. The trail led first to the optician who had made the glasses, but he had filled similar prescriptions for thousands of people. The frames, however, weren't quite as ordinary as they looked. In one small detail they differed from the others. The hinge connecting the earpiece to the nosepiece was patented, manufactured by a single optical company in Rochester, New York, and sold in Chicago by only one outlet, which had handled this kind of frame for only a few months. During that time, as a matter of fact, it had sold just three of those frames. One was for a lawyer, who happened to have been in Europe at the time of the murder. Another belonged to a woman who readily produced her glasses. The third pair of frames belonged to Leopold.

Since the crime they planned was going to be perfect, Leopold and Loeb had rehearsed an alibi—just in case some minor hitch occurred. When they were called for questioning, they trotted out their story. On May 24, they told the police, they had picked up a couple of girls in Leopold's car and driven them out to Lincoln Park. But their alibi was quickly shot down by the Leopold family chauffeur, who said that the car had not been out of the garage that day.

They had admitted being together, and the glasses tied Leopold to the scene of the crime. As if that weren't enough, tests indicated that the ransom note had been written on a typewriter owned by one of them. Their arrest followed immediately. The case against them appeared to be solid. The one question remaining as far as the public was concerned was: would they be executed? Robert E. Crowe, the Illinois State Attorney, had moved quickly for an indictment for kidnapping and murder, and he made it clear that he would demand the death sentence.

The plea of not guilty by reason of insanity, available to defendants since the middle of the nineteenth century, was always a possibility for them, although Leopold, at the time, immediately discounted that avenue of escape. "I thought...I'm not crazy," he later recalled. "I know the legal definition of insanity: inability to distinguish between right and wrong. How can we possibly fall under that definition? So there's no problem about insanity here."

The families spared no expense to save their offspring. They engaged Clarence Darrow, probably the most famous lawyer in America and a prominent opponent of capital punishment. Crowe was certain that Darrow would opt for the insanity defense, but hoped that widespread public horror at the "thrill-killing" aspect of the crime, with which the newspapers were having a field day, would carry the jury.

Darrow, however, was also aware of the atmosphere in which the trial would be conducted. When the proceedings opened, he stunned the courtroom by announcing that his clients would not plead insanity, that they would admit responsibility for their crime. They would rely, he stated, on the mercy of the court. Darrow had sidestepped the need for a jury; he would play only to the judge—*who would decide whether they would live or die.* Crowe felt enraged and defrauded. He called for a delay to better prepare the state's case, which Judge John R. Caverly granted.

On July 24, 1924, the trial got under way. Crowe wasn't taking any chances of being outfoxed by the wily Darrow. He called 102 witnesses to pound home the idea that the murder of Bobby Franks had been a cold-blooded, premeditated crime, committed by young men in full possession of their faculties.

But the gray-haired sixty-seven-year-old Darrow had not earned his reputation for nothing. The boys would not formally plead insanity, but that didn't mean they couldn't arrive at the same end from a different direction. During

those hot summer weeks before the trial, Darrow had employed five of the country's leading psychiatrists to prepare a complete examination of his clients—not to
demonstrate that they were insane, which he had already
disclaimed, but to show what their family lives had been
like, and how they had lived in the society of which they
were part.

First, Karl Bowman and Harold Hulbert inquired into
their family background, interviewed their friends and
examined the prisoners themselves. With their report as
a basis, three other psychiatrists conducted their own examinations—William A. White; William Healy, who had
begun Chicago's Juvenile Court, one of the first in the
country; and Bernard Glueck, an expert in criminal psy-
chopathology, with long experience among the inmates
of Sing Sing Prison.

Dr. White was to be the first witness for the defense,
and Crowe sought to block his testimony. The prosecutor
claimed that White was trying to establish a case for a
kind of moral insanity, and that the court should not permit it. But the judge wanted to hear him out, and his
decision opened the door to the development of Darrow's
case.

Now, in a masterly presentation, Darrow had the psychiatrists lay out systematically, in detail, the private
lives of both Leopold and Loeb—their homosexuality, the
king/slave relationship and all that followed from it.

In his oft-quoted summation, Darrow focused on
whether or not a society should react to violence with its
own violence. "Cruelty only breeds cruelty, hatred only
causes hatred," he told the judge. "Do I need to argue that
if there is any way to soften this human heart, which is

hard at best; if there is any way to kill evil and hatred and all that goes with it, it is not through evil and hatred and cruelty? It is through charity and love and understanding. How often do people need to be told this? Look back at the world. There is not a philosopher, not a religious leader, not a creed that has not taught it.

"In truth," Darrow went on, now getting to the essence of his speech, "I am not pleading so much for these boys as I am for the infinite number of others to follow, those who perhaps cannot be so well defended as these." Then, looking directly at Judge Caverly, he concluded: "Men and women who do not think will applaud you if you send these boys to their death. I know Your Honor stands between the future and the past. I know the future is with me and what I stand for here. I do not know how much salvage there is in these two boys. I hate to say it in their presence, but what is there to look forward to? I do not know but what Your Honor would be merciful if you tied a rope around their necks and let them die; merciful to them, but not merciful to civilization and not merciful to those who would be left behind."

The judge gathered up his papers and went into seclusion for two weeks while he prepared his decision. When the court reconvened, on September 19, 1924, he announced: "It would have been the path of least resistance to impose the extreme penalty of the law..." Then he added, "You are both sentenced to life imprisonment and ninety-nine years for kidnapping." He duly noted the reports of the five psychiatrists as a valuable contribution to criminology, but this approach to the criminal mind— which circumvented the familiar not-guilty-by-reason-of-insanity plea—was more worthy of legislative than of

53

judicial consideration. The reports had not affected his decision.

In giving Leopold and Loeb life in prison instead of sending them to the gallows, Judge Caverly cited his belief that "to the offenders, particularly of the type they are, the prolonged suffering of years of confinement may well be the severer form of retribution and expiation." Leopold saw the overriding irony in it. "If Judge Caverly meant literally what he said in his opinion," he later wrote, "the whole elaborate psychiatric defense presented in our behalf and the herculean efforts of our brilliant counsel were of no avail. The only thing that influenced him to choose imprisonment instead of death was our youth; we need only have introduced our birth certificates in evidence!"

One other aspect of the decision—and Judge Caverly's state of mind—deserves comment. His review of the case was curious, and it reflected, perhaps, more of the current state of American manners and mores than it did of the specifics of Darrow's presentation and the evidence that was available. Throughout the trial, the subject of sex had been stifled, as if it were a decidedly unwelcome interloper in Judge Caverly's courtroom. When sex raised its ugly head, the attorneys had been asked to approach the bench, and interchanges were carried on in a whisper.

But the defendants' sexuality and their feelings about it had everything to do with the matter at hand. Leopold and Loeb's homosexuality had been established by a fraternity brother, who had witnessed them making love. The fact that the Franks boy had been found naked from the waist down and the nature of the psychological profile of the two defendants strongly suggested a sexual dimension to the crime. Their homosexuality certainly did not of itself imply pederasty and necrophilia, but their particular personalities and the available physical evidence suggested that the young boy's body had been sexually abused. Yet the judge expressed his conviction that the evidence was "conclusive" that "there was no abuse offered to the body of the victim." Perhaps he found the very possibility that such a thing might have happened too repugnant to contemplate. (Leopold, incidentally, maintained to his dying day that Bobby Franks had not been sexually molested.)

III

Why did they do it? Why does anybody commit murder for "thrills"? Was it senseless?

We naturally recoil in horror when an act of violence is committed for which there does not seem to be a discernible motive. But unconscious motives make sense to the unconscious mind. The mind has its reasons—coherent, systematic and rational. There is a "logic" to even the strangest pattern of behavior, even if the person within whom the behavior maintains consistency seems totally mad to outsiders. The murder committed by these two young men—boys, really—was horrible, an outrage against everything we think of as civilized. But in the context of their psychic development, it made a good deal of sense.

To be young and a homosexual in the early 1920s was to live a life of damnation. There was no support from a gay community, no sense that one might be just following an alternative life-style. Some people might be able to handle the closeted existence demanded by such realities, but not Leopold and Loeb. They were very much aware that by the standards of their time, they felt decidedly "abnormal." Whatever bravado they manifested in their fantasies and plans, their self-images were those of men who were degraded by their sexuality.

The product of this gap between what they were and what they felt they should have been was an abiding, tormenting sense of guilt. Loeb, especially, was obsessed by guilt to a point at which he was suicidal. The corollary of the guilt feelings was a deep-seated need for punishment. In small ways we all manifest this phenomenon in our lives, but Leopold and Loeb carried it to a murderous extreme.

In killing Bobby Franks, Loeb was, in a sense, attempting to commit a kind of indirect suicide. His grandiose and childish fantasy of being the master criminal committing the perfect crime notwithstanding, he had a strong inner need to be caught and—most likely—executed. We know from those who observed him in prison that he seemed almost joyous over his incarceration. It was a fulfillment of the jail fantasy he had toyed with since childhood. It may have been the only place that could ever have made him happy.

Nathan Leopold was motivated by both his own sense of guilt and his sexual subjugation to Richard Loeb. His rush to leave the scene of the crime certainly suggests a not altogether comfortable feeling about what they were doing. He was in such a hurry to get away that he dropped his topcoat—which, as it happened, held the glasses that finally incriminated him. The fact of his losing the glasses may or may not have been mere chance—we can never know for sure. But given the guilt feelings about his sexuality, we could speculate that he too had a desire to be caught.

Leopold's total attachment to his friend made his complicity inevitable. "My motive, so far as I can be said to have had one," he later observed, "was to please Dick. Just that—incredible as it sounds. I thought so much of the guy that I was willing to do anything—even commit murder—if he wanted it bad enough. And he wanted to do this—very badly indeed."

Both Leopold and Loeb were sent to the Illinois State Penitentiary to spend the rest of their lives. The "execution" that Judge Caverly had spared them finally caught up to Loeb in 1936 while he was taking a bath. He was cut to pieces with a razor by another inmate. But Leopold lived on, and in time developed the hope that he might still be able to make something of his life.

In 1949, at the age of forty-four, Nathan Leopold made a plea for parole, but he was turned down. In 1955, the parole board, considering another of his applications for release from prison, asked me for my opinion. On the basis of what I knew at the time—and in retrospect, I think I should have made an effort to know more—I told them that it would be premature to let him out.

In 1957, he made still another plea for his freedom. His lawyer, Elmer Gertz, wrote to me stating that "We are particularly eager to hear from you on the basis of your personal knowledge of Nathan Leopold. We are trying to give a complete picture of the situation derived from the recollections and impressions of those like yourself who have been in personal contact with him at any time during his more than 33 years of imprisonment." Leopold had fond memories of our conversations in 1941, and he hoped that at this juncture I might be able to say something in his behalf.

I gave the matter lengthy consideration. I asked to see his record, and I discovered that he had been an exemplary prisoner. During World War II he had volunteered to be a guinea pig for experiments aimed at finding a cure for malaria. He had also established a correspondence school for fellow prisoners. In every sense he gave evidence of having become a man whose behavior belied the antisocial traits he had manifested as a youth. I was reminded, too, that he had not been the actual killer, only an accomplice. Thirty-three years seemed long enough to atone for that.

But far more important, I felt, was to determine whether the problems growing out of his homosexuality might still get him into trouble. At this stage in his life, it seemed to me, his sexual drive had diminished to a point at which it was no longer likely to overshadow his good judgment. I finally concluded that his lawyer had been correct when he wrote to me that Nathan Leopold had "been sufficiently punished, is remorseful, has been fully rehabilitated, and is in no sense a menace to society."

In March 1958, after thirty-four years of incarceration, Nathan Leopold walked out of prison. The now middle-aged man, wearing "a new prison-made blue suit, $639.33 in his pocket" with a "grey herring-bone overcoat" to ward off the early-spring chill, was besieged by a swarm of photographers and reporters. A condition of his parole had been that he would avoid the limelight—and privacy was also what he himself desired. He had prepared a statement:

Among you are men and women I count my personal friends. Many of you—I hope all of you—feel that a third of a century spent in prison has been severe punishment and are happy to see me free.

I hope you want to see me succeed, to see me vindicate the trust reposed in me.

Don't, then, I beg you, add to that punishment; don't make it impossible for me to succeed.

I appeal as solemnly as I know how to you, and to your editors, and to your publishers, and to society at large, to agree that the only piece of news about me is that I have ceased to be news.

I beg, I beseech you and your editors and your publishers to grant me a gift almost as precious as freedom itself—a gift without which freedom ceases to have much value— the gift of privacy.

Give me a chance—a fair chance—to start life anew.

They did. It was a one-day story.

Leopold found a job in Puerto Rico, as a laboratory technician in a hospital operated by the Church of the Brethren, about eighty miles from San Juan. A year later he wrote to me, describing his happiness with his job and the people he worked with. He continued to do well, and later married.

In January 1966, I met him once more, for the last time, when I was invited to give a lecture at the University of San Juan. Lova and I saw him and his wife, Trudi, at our hotel and had a long talk. He was as bright and knowledgeable as when I had first encountered him many years before. The only difference—aside from the fact that he had obviously aged—was the light in his eyes when he talked about being free.

He asked me what I was going to lecture about, and when I told him the subject was murder, he said that he wanted to hear my talk. That surprised me. I thought he might have had his fill of the topic. He came, nevertheless, entering just before I began, nodding to me as he sat down in the first row. As I spoke I could see his face, serious and intent, but showing no other emotion. Afterward he came up to me, told me he had enjoyed the talk, shook my hand and left quietly.

Nathan Leopold died in Puerto Rico in 1974, from a combination of diabetes and heart and kidney disease. The world had not forgotten him—who could forget the story of two brilliant youths who had used their unusual abilities to commit what they thought would be the perfect crime, and had brought ruin and disgrace to themselves and their families? It was a tragedy that touched more than one life. But Nathan Leopold's return to society had also shown that a person can be salvaged even against the worst odds.

3
SELF-EXECUTION THROUGH MURDER

Eighteen-year-old Harvey had been arrested for a series of robberies of young women. While committing his crime he would always tie up his victim, and often touch her body, but did not carry the sexual act further. He said he got an erection when he did this, although he did not ejaculate.

When I interviewed Harvey for the first time, I noted that he was slight and appeared to be shorter than he actually was. His manner was effeminate. (This was of particular concern to the authorities, because there was always the danger that he would be viewed as sexual prey by bigger and older men in the prison.) His face was covered with pimples, and he always looked down instead of straight at me; he seemed to be constantly ashamed, as if he wanted to apologize for his existence. He stammered, and often bit his fingernails.

Harvey seemed to find it almost unbearable to talk about

61

himself. After much probing, he told me that he had few friends, liked to play the guitar and ran for exercise. Although he liked school, especially math and science, his interest had waned when he began to get into trouble.

When I asked him what was bothering him, he mentioned, after some hesitation, that he had never been able to ask a girl for a date; he was just too shy. Then he told me that since the age of seven or eight he had thought of himself as a woman hater. He was often depressed, and as he got older he frequently fantasized about committing suicide. "I almost hanged myself at age eleven," he told me in a high-pitched, timid voice. "I had a rope and was fooling around to see what it felt like." When I asked him why he wanted to die, he became evasive. This pattern would recur often in our conversations. First he would offer some information; then he would become silent, preoccupied, secretive. It was clear to me, even at the beginning of my acquaintance with him, that Harvey's depression, suicidal fantasies and aborted suicide attempt expressed self-hatred and marked feelings of guilt.

Harvey viewed his father as aggressive, punitive and domineering. He had a vivid memory of being caught masturbating by him more than once and being beaten with his father's belt, with the added warning that self-stimulation would drive him crazy and rot his brain. Harvey's pimples were a direct consequence of masturbation, he recalled his father telling him, and they revealed his habit to the whole world. Furthermore, his father cautioned, every time the boy did it he would lose a pint of blood.

Although Harvey feared his father, he expressed love for his mother, even though he felt that she rejected him.

She too appeared to be afraid of his father. In fact, she was afraid to discuss the man with us other than to say that she was forced to submit to his domineering and controlling nature; she offered Harvey no bulwark against him.

In his first major crime, Harvey held up a woman with a toy pistol. In the course of the robbery, he tied her hands and feet with string, loosened her dress and touched her breast. Then he left her without doing anything else. I got no reply when I asked him if he was afraid to go further with his sexual advances.

In subsequent crimes, he used a real pistol that he found in an apartment he burglarized; and he continued the pattern of tying up his victims. In one incident he described to me, he tied a woman's hands and then walked her outside of town to the side of a hill, where they spent the night. He finally fell asleep and in the morning took her back into the town and released her. It is not clear why she did not leave when he was asleep; perhaps, as is often the case with hostages, the victim may have temporarily identified with her captor.

In the few months after his high school graduation Harvey was arrested several times for theft, although he was treated with leniency because of his youth and intelligence.

He was paroled in the custody of his parents, but soon ran away and reverted to his now familiar criminal pattern. The next time he was arrested he was sent to the Reception Center for Youthful Offenders, where the psychiatrists who evaluated him reported that "Unless he receives intensive psychotherapy, it is not likely that the correctional institution will improve his deep-seated personality difficulties, which make him potentially a dangerous individual at large."

Dr. Milton Berger of Stony Lodge Hospital in Ossining, who had examined Harvey, knew about my work in a research project on sex offenders at Sing Sing. Our aim, innovative for its time, was to probe the conscious and unconscious motivations for sex-related crimes and develop means of treatment. But Berger's specific concern was to solicit my advice on what might be done with Harvey. At my suggestion the boy, who was under sentencing, was transferred to the prison, which is where I began my work with him.

In our initial interviews, Harvey, although he was not psychotic, was clearly having trouble maintaining full contact with reality. He recognized the bizarre nature of his behavior, but could not accept it. I believe that for him, taking money from his victims appeared to be not so much a matter of stealing as a means for gratifying his sexual needs, which he could not bring himself to do in the customary fashion. Gradually, he began to see this.

In evaluating the case I also examined his parents. As time went on, the conflicted family relationships gradually became clearer. Outwardly, Harvey was in many ways the dutiful son. He feared his father and expressed love for his mother, although he felt she rejected him. But inwardly he was in rebellion, which made him feel very guilty. In the dynamics of this family, the father dominated the wife, and she in turn controlled the son. Caught in a bind—terribly unhappy but feeling powerless to give vent to his emotions—Harvey had become passive and depressed. Under the psychological pounding he had been taking from his father, Harvey had long since come to doubt his own masculinity; indeed, he felt emasculated. He had severe guilt feelings about sex. Perceiving himself to be totally inadequate and incapable of approaching women in a socially acceptable way, he sought to resolve his problem by literally overpowering and controlling them.

Sing Sing was hardly a country club; it was bound to have taken a toll on him. Inmates in adjoining cells were always having loud conversations, often about sex, a subject that naturally caused Harvey a great deal of anxiety. Nor did his father's visits help the young man's peace of mind. In view of the stressful situation and his history of suicidal fantasies, a close watch was kept on him.

For some time Harvey had been having nightmares that revealed strong but unconscious incestuous feelings toward his mother. His intense rivalry with his father and his desire to possess and dominate his mother, whom he obviously could not have, were being vividly and frighteningly played out in his dream world. Finally the pressure built up to the point where the unbearable conflict could no longer be kept in the realm of sleep.

One night I was called and told that Harvey had been screaming and threatening to take his life. But when I got to the prison and spoke to him, he was composed, and he told me that any suicidal thoughts he might have had were "gone." At least for the moment. He related that he had always harbored desire for both life and death, but that now the life force was dominant. He thought he saw signs of improvement and felt that he was gaining greater insight into himself. I sought to reassure him that he was getting good treatment, and by the end of the interview he seemed quite cheerful. Nevertheless, I instructed the psychiatrist on duty at the prison that Harvey should be watched closely, and if he experienced similar periods of disturbance, he should be sedated and transferred to the prison's isolation ward. I also convinced the warden that Harvey's regular cell should be in a quieter part of the prison, so as to reduce the general level of stress he was feeling.

Harvey made slow progress. Gradually he became aware of how his feelings of rejection had colored his life. He began to realize how self-absorbed he was and began to gain some insight into the way his behavior toward everyone reflected the manner in which he dealt with his parents. He had learned only one way to get what he wanted; mope or grunt or fret to make others feel guilty unless they satisfied his needs.

But despite signs of improvement, it became clear in the second year of treatment that he was still unable to resolve his conflicts. Unconsciously, Harvey blamed and resented his mother for rejecting him, and had contempt for her passive acceptance of his father's harshness and domination. Consciously, though, he continued to feel that his own inadequacy caused her to reject him. So his buried hatred of his mother surfaced in his behavior toward other women, in the particular pattern of his crime. And despite his increasing ability to recognize, at least on an intellectual level, how his image of women had been distorted, he still found it difficult to relate that to his tying them up.

The irony of his criminal pattern was that he was "tying up" himself along with the women. In making them helpless, Harvey was imitating his father's treatment of his mother, which he unconsciously found stimulating. But he was also tying up the mother who had frustrated him, and he was saying to her, "Look, Mother. I am tying you up. I don't want you, but you are not going to get me either." Where did that leave him? Spitefully impotent, guilty and self-punishing.

One of the barriers to real change in Harvey's condition was his attitude toward authority, which he had derived from his relationship with his father. He mistrusted all of us in the sex-offender research project, sometimes expressing feelings that were actually paranoid. If anything, his resistance grew, and he continued to feel that everyone found him ridiculous. He remained careful not to reveal too much of himself, and rarely emerged from his shell.

As time passed, we often discussed the possibility of having him transferred to a mental hospital for more intensive treatment. But we rejected this because we assumed that if he were kept at Sing Sing until paroled, we would be in a better position to see to it that he remained under observation for many years after his release—which in his case seemed to be a prudent step.

As the time drew near when Harvey would first be eligible for parole, he had a dream that seemed to reflect several matters which concerned him. In it he found himself standing between two buildings talking very freely to another person. In the past he had usually been able to free-associate from the subject matter of his dreams—that is, he was able to let his mind wander after relating a dream and say whatever came into his head. But this time it proved to be a little harder. Finally, when asked what the two buildings might mean, he mentioned that they reminded him of a woman's legs. This was a powerful and overwhelming image—he could have been squashed by a woman with such legs.

Aside from expressing his fear of women, the dream

also suggested that he had ambivalent feelings about his upcoming meeting with the parole board. In talking freely to another person he was saying that he was ready to get out of Sing Sing; but in putting himself in a position between a woman's enormous legs, he was also expressing feelings of helplessness. Consciously he wanted to be released; the staff psychiatrists, however, felt that he was not yet ready for freedom.

He felt angry and frustrated when the parole board gave him one more year. Shortly afterward, he had a dream that he was on a platform and that many obstacles obstructed his view. One of the obstacles was a new law concerning sex offenders which, in fact, had already been enacted at my suggestion; Harvey had recently learned about it (It took effect April 1, 1950). The law provided indeterminate sentences of one year to life for persons convicted of sexual offenses, the final length of the imprisonment to be determined by the prisoner's mental condition. Every half-year the offender would be given another psychiatric examination to see if he was fit for release. Harvey was aware enough of the compulsive character of his behavior to think that the new law could spell trouble for him.

He was beginning to dream about getting out of prison, but even in his dream world things did not always go smoothly. In one dream, for example, the guards were opening the cell doors, but when they came to his they passed it by. It was a nightmare from which he woke up screaming. Paranoid feelings still undermined his fragile ego.

In the next few months, however, at least on the surface, Harvey seemed to be growing more at peace with himself and demonstrated a better understanding of his problems. New psychological tests indicated that he had more conscious control of his motives and impulses. Yet there were still signs of an ego that had been severely buffeted.

At the next parole-board meeting in December 1950, Harvey was advised that he would be paroled in a month. I asked him at that time to write about his feelings and his situation, and he wrote:

> Frankly, I feel kind of happy and tired. Happy because I will soon be going home and a turning point in my life has been reached where I believe that the future years will be much more pleasant and happy than the last ones. I am tired because for a long number of years I have been waging quite a battle to understand and conquer the deficiencies and fears which for too many years became an integral part of my personality and led to much unhappiness and ultimately to jail. I'm very grateful...I feel myself quite sure that by continuing the process of self-understanding when I return to a normal physical environment (that is when I get out of jail) that I will be able to live a happy life and in some small way be useful in this world.

A few months later, Harvey was paroled in the custody of his parents on the condition that he continue psychiatric treatment. Harvey was still a troubled young man, and he would not find it easy to deal with the stress and strain of the outside world and needed every break he could get. I was not happy that he was returning to the same family situation that had fostered his criminal mentality in the first place.

But our staff no longer had any say in the matter—and once Harvey was released, our worst fears were realized.

69

The parole supervision was not strict. His parents soon left the state, and we lost touch with the boy. We could only hope that he would continue in treatment wherever he was, and that he would continue to gain in self-control and self-esteem and develop a more positive attitude toward life.

Seven years later, while in California on research, I opened the newspaper one morning and saw on the front page a story about a young man who had been arrested for strangling three women. Before killing them he had tied them up with string. This is Harvey, I thought with dread; this is something he would have done. Sadly, I was right. Under the pretext of seeking models to photograph, he had, on three separate occasions, taken the women outside Los Angeles and murdered them.

Later I learned from Dr. Bernard Diamond, who examined him at this time, that Harvey was relieved to have been caught and had confessed quite readily to the crimes. I was not surprised when he took no measures to defend himself. Given his strong sense of guilt and suicidal feelings, there was only one way out in his scheme of things: to die.

At his trial he pleaded guilty and was sentenced to death. His lawyer and Dr. Diamond urged him repeatedly to ask for clemency, but Harvey refused to sign the request.

It was a sad drama that was being acted out in California. Three young women had had to die for Harvey to act out his fantasies. Narcissistic and infantile even now, he was showing his contempt for authority by daring the state to execute him. And he was reveling in the national attention he drew. His strenuous objections to clemency resulted in front-page stories about "the young man who prefers death to life." His ego was flattered; the limelight was his. At last Harvey was a hero.

Most people who kill harbor the seeds of self-destruction. Like Harvey, Richard Loeb, for example, was gripped by tensions that could have pushed him either way; as it happens, his circumstances favored the projection of his rage outward. But even with Loeb, the ultimate unconscious aim may have been the death of the self, for despite his pretensions to criminal perfection, he knew that there was a good chance he would be caught and possibly executed.

But I felt there was a further dimension to Harvey. The public bravado was being trumpeted against a quiet backdrop of ambivalence. His very defiance was also an unconscious manifestation of his will to live. Yet now, ironically, he was finally to have more control over the course of his life than he had ever had—by forcing his own death. And when he finally inhaled the fumes of the gas chamber, the state helped him to become the master of his fate.

4
THE NICEST GUY
IN BALTIMORE

On a June evening in 1957, tall, elegantly hand-
some and socially prominent Robert Jett Van Horn found
himself holding the battered, bloody and half-nude body
of his wife, Bernice. As far as he could recall, he had
beaten her with his fists in an uncontrollable rage after
she had hit him on the head with her handbag during an
argument. His memory was rather hazy about the details.

Rarely had Baltimore's criminal court seen such a mon-
eyed audience. The gossip among the women was of the
latest cotillion. The defendant's seventy-nine-year-old
parents arrived at the courthouse every day in a Cadillac
limousine driven by their chauffeur. When Van Horn's
brother was informed of the trouble, he had to be called
off the famed, exclusive Burning Tree golf course in a
suburb of Washington. Robert Van Horn, lumber and real
estate executive, was, as fourteen of his rich and well-
placed friends testifying as character witnesses swore, "the

nicest guy in Baltimore...the nicest man on earth," an individual who "wouldn't harm a fly." They thought the world of him; and they seemed to have enjoyed his company at lunch so frequently that, from their testimony, one would suspect he ate lunch twenty times a week.

There was no doubt that the fifty-five-year-old Baltimore aristocrat had killed his wife; but his state of mind, his intentions and thus his ultimate culpability were yet to be determined.

Van Horn's stress and confusion were evident in the rambling statement he gave to the police two days after the murder, from which this is excerpted:

> On Saturday evening, June 1, after attending a party, my wife and I drove to our farm on Falls Road above Shawan, which we often did on nice evenings. We drove in, talked to Mr. Straw the farmer, observed the beautiful moon...
>
> We had never lived at the farm, but she had been against considering it. We lighted up the whole house, went over it and got into a discussion about living out there. My point was that other people could get along without a servant for two people, and that made her argue...I'm afraid she thought I was making direct criticism of her when I talked about the fact that two people ought to be able to get along without domestic help in short periods of time, at least. One word led to another, but without real animus until we were out on the porch in the dark going to the car.
>
> I was walking down the steps ahead, also she could see them, when she made a sharp remark. I turned over my shoulder and I suppose replied in kind. We were in the dark except for whatever moonlight was there, and I didn't see her swing her evening bag at me; knocked my glasses and stung me sharply. I went into the only red rage I ever remember having. I don't know what I hit her with except

my fists, but the first thing I knew was the farmer calling to ask if everything was all right. I told him "Yes," which couldn't have been wronger—she was dead.

I sat there with her head in my lap for several hours— I don't know how long. I then placed her in the front seat with me and started to leave. The time might be determined from the tenant farmer who passed me on the driveway— he was coming in. I drove around all over the country into the city and back trying to decide what to do—in a complete daze. Around dawn I felt that the only course was to destroy myself. After making that decision, I placed her body where I later informed the police they could find it, went to my apartment, changed my clothes and went to my office to make various personal arrangements in anticipation of destroying myself. I didn't want the shirt and suit to be around the apartment, even though I didn't expect to be there myself. I threw the suit and shirt in the water off Waterview Avenue.

I went to my office and proceeded with various personal arrangements. When they were completed, I drove out to the farm about four P.M. intending to tell Mr. Straw what I was going to do, but he was not there. I then returned to my wife's body and stayed there until the police arrived. . . . When leaving the apartment on Greenway, I took with me the clothes that were bloodstained and soaked the shirt with water to remove bloodstains from the seat. While at the office I changed shoes, and when leaving the office I took along the remnants of a bottle of whiskey and the gun I intended to use to destroy myself. While at the office I called my brother, Charles R. Van Horn, in Washington, D.C., and told him what had taken place.

On a memorandum pad in his station wagon, the police had found notes making further reference to the murder. Here Van Horn had written: "*Good bye darling wherever you are please believe that I am desolate at losing you and heart broken that I made it so. If only you had eased off once in a while! I humored you, babied you and went far out of my way to keep you happy because you were, I thought, fundamentally a simple and quiet girl. You have lately become complicated in a simple but perverse way."* At the lumber company where he was an executive, the authorities discovered another letter written to the police, again describing the crime. Here he concluded his account of the incidents of June 1 with: *"My anguish at what I have done is boundless and though I truly did not know what I was doing until too late, I must be punished. May God rest her lovely soul and may He in his wisdom find means to forgive my horrible act of violence."*

John Grayson Turnbull, a shrewd and articulate former state senator, had been engaged to defend Van Horn. His strategy was to convince the court that his client had not been possessed of his full faculties when he committed the crime against his fifty-year-old wife. The defense would be based on the M'Naghten Rule, derived from the British legal system; it is still the yardstick by which criminal insanity is judged in several states. The M'Naghten Rule states: "To establish a defense on the ground of insanity, it must be clearly proved that at the time of the act the accused was laboring under such a defect of reasoning as not to know the nature and quality of his act, or, if he did, that he did not know that what he was doing was wrong." Quickly Turnbull rounded up the best doctors in Baltimore—foremost among them the well-known psychiatrist Manfred Guttmacher, whom I had known for several years. When Turnbull asserted that Van Horn had been insane when he killed his wife, the media immediately played up his contention with great fanfare.

The prosecution would be directed by the young district attorney of Towson, Maryland, Frank H. Newell III. Newell was no amateur. He had worked on a number of cases involving extreme violence, and had already been written up in *Life* magazine for his ingenious detective work in solving one particularly difficult and important murder case. He asked one of the Manhattan assistant district attorneys to approach me about entering the case as an expert witness for the state, and I found the facts of the case—as they were known so far—to be intriguing.

My job, as usual, would be to examine the defendant, present a written report to the court with my observations and conclusions as to Van Horn's state of mind when the crime was committed and be available for testimony during the trial.

I examined Van Horn on five different occasions, spending altogether about nine hours with him, two of them with Dr. Israel Wechsler, one of the country's most renowned neurologists.

Van Horn looked older than his fifty-five years. He spoke slowly, in a subdued voice, without evincing any emotion except that of depression—which was not unreasonable, since he was about to go on trial for murder. He was well spoken, and his bearing was dignified. Sometimes when he spoke, tears came to his eyes and he looked toward me as if he were asking for help. He was cooperative throughout the interviews until I would ask him directly about the murder. He would react as if he had been rudely awakened, and say in a determined voice: "I don't remember."

There was an interesting aspect of this crime that did

not surface publicly until Van Horn's trial was well under way. The coroner's report described injuries to Bernice Van Horn which indicated clearly that she had been run over by an automobile. Van Horn seemed to have no memory of this having happened.

His memory, of course, was central to the case. He might or might not have been selective with his recollections. He had already been examined by several other psychiatrists and by now could have developed routine answers to sticky questions. His honesty on that account remained to be seen.

The district attorney told me about Van Horn's family background. His father, a retired executive vice-president of the Baltimore & Ohio Railroad, was outgoing, while his mother was more withdrawn, although her son was later to assure me of her marked intelligence. Van Horn's brother, Charles, forty-nine years old, was married but childless. He too was an executive of the B&O Railroad. There was also a sister who had died.

He identified with both his sister and his mother, rather than his father. His mother had been overprotective, rewarding his passive dependency at the time when he should have been developing some independence necessary for successful functioning in the adult world. Where there should have been self-confidence and a general openness to life, Van Horn had been left with anxiety, timidity and fear.

In one of our sessions, Van Horn mentioned, somewhat reluctantly, a recent dream. "I saw her," he related. "I had the feeling of forgiveness. I saw my wife."

He was more than willing to talk about Bernice. Although he made an effort to appear gallant when discussing his wife, his bluntly critical attitude toward her kept breaking through. She had been jealous, occasionally alienating his friends. She had been "afraid of psychiatry, of mental illness" and had seemed to have a phobia about mental hospitals. Once, when they were going to visit a patient at a mental institution, he had had to turn the car around and drive back because of her intense reaction when she saw the place.

Bernice had also been obsessed with death. She had had a phobia about cemeteries; she had never visited her mother's grave, and she did not attend funerals. She had always thought she was at death's door, probably already harboring a deadly cancer. One of her pet obsessions had been her knuckle—she thought it was growing bigger, being consumed by a tumor. "I never expressed anger before," he remarked of his reaction to her peculiarities before the night of the murder. "When she got hysterical," he recalled, "all I did was comfort her."

Bernice had been widowed in 1951, and after her first husband's death she had begun to drink. "If she didn't have a drink she was upset. So we carried whiskey with us, to have on the road," Van Horn recounted. He spoke of himself as a moderate drinker. I tried to turn the conversation back to Van Horn himself. I asked him why he had not married until the age of fifty-two. He said he had had more than enough girlfriends in his life. Indeed, he boasted of his active sex life. On the other hand, he acknowledged, when he had started masturbating at age thirteen, he had had to be shown how by a farm boy. This suggested to me that he had at least some ambivalence, if not fear, about sex; his late marriage also brought up the possibility that his attitude toward women in general was mixed.

He spoke of his concern, as a youth, for the salvation

of his soul, suggesting a twisted religious passion that bordered on the morbid. "When I was thirteen years old," he told me, "I lived in a little town, Olina, Ohio. We had a revival meeting. I was taken with a feeling of great sin. It went on for some months. I used to fall down on my knees in the street and pray, like a compulsion." He described the feeling of depression this had left him with. He had become obsessed with sin, and had been afraid that his father "would go to hell" for having not repented of *his* sins.

All this talk of sin led me to ask him if he had felt personal guilt. "About customary sin—sex," he replied. "I masturbated often—three, four times a week. That was part of my sin."

Shortly after that, he began to speak of a series of illnesses he had suffered as a young man. In 1922 he had had typhoid fever followed by pneumonia. In the spring of 1923 he had contracted gonorrhea from the wife of the history teacher at the school he was attending. In 1926 he had developed tuberculosis and had spent a long stretch in a sanatorium, where, he claimed, he had "had sex...with the female patients."

Of all the illnesses Van Horn mentioned, the only one that had any real bearing on his case was a malady that had originally been attributed to Mona, his sister. She had had a very unhappy marriage and drank a great deal. She had died in 1955, at the age of forty-eight, shortly after spending three months in a sanatorium drying out. It was not her alcoholism, however, that was crucial to an understanding of Van Horn's thoughts and actions on the night of June 1, but rather the defense's contention that Mona had had epilepsy as well and that it ran in the family. Van Horn claimed that epilepsy had influenced him on the night of the murder.

Van Horn's memory, or lack of it, about the murder was a problem. While I did not think he was simply lying, I did not have the feeling that this was an actual case of amnesia, or loss of memory, brought on by epilepsy. It seemed to be more a matter of repression of painful memories.

I questioned how Van Horn could have suffered from epilepsy if he had never been under a doctor's care for it. An electroencephalogram that had recently been done on him indicated a normal pattern of brain waves—although in fairness, about 15 percent of such tests done on true epileptics will show the same result.

The crux of the matter was the exact nature of his sister's illness: was it genuine epilepsy, or had her symptoms been caused by something else? We decided to subpoena her hospital records.

There were, it turns out, ten doctors on the side of the prosecution and ten who would speak for the defense— two small medical armies about to face each other in battle. Dr. Guttmacher headed up the experts for the defense, and I was in charge of the group for the prosecution. As in some medieval court intrigue, loyalties were in a state of flux. One psychiatrist engaged by the defense had already come over to the side of the prosecution, having finally concluded that Van Horn had not been insane at the time he killed his wife.

Rumors and speculation were beginning to run rampant. Some thought that money might have been the motivation for the killing. It was also rumored that the defense attorney had already been offered a quarter of a million dollars if he could get his client off the hook.

I had other things on my mind. There was still work to be done in examining Robert Jett Van Horn.

I knew that it was time for me to find out from Van Horn, as best he could tell me, or as far as he was willing to reveal, what exactly had happened on the night of the murder. When I asked him to describe the course of events, he repeated to me what he had already told the police. He looked away and tried to hide his face when he spoke.

I asked if he had felt hatred at the time he killed his wife. "It must have been more hatred than I could feel," he replied. If he lived "to be a hundred," he said, he would "never forget the way she looked." Then he described getting out a flashlight to check her pulse—a fairly involved procedure for someone supposedly in something of a trance. He related how he had cleaned up afterward and then proceeded to write a number of letters—to the police, his brother and a minister. The next day he had called his brother and told him what had happened and that he was going to kill himself. The brother had tried to talk him out of suicide, but at this point Robert had been adamant.

After a few drinks, Van Horn had called the police and reported his wife's death. When they arrived, he was sitting in his car holding a .32 revolver, with which, he said, he intended to shoot himself. At that point, he told me, "The detective dived into the car and grabbed the gun....I still think I would have done it. Something held me back. Maybe we all want to live, to justify. Nobody wants to do it. Maybe I was trying to justify some reason why I should live."

"What happened at her burial?" I asked.

"The following Tuesday I was in shock; the funeral arrangements were turned over to a friend, a distant cousin. Bernice's father died when she was nine or ten years old; her mother died in 1948 or '49. They didn't have the courtesy to invite my parents [to Bernice's funeral]. It was held privately. My brother was invited; he went."

At that point, he described his situation as a "bad dream." I thought that his answer to my question was evasive and that it expressed feelings that seemed less than appropriate to the occasion. He seemed determined to focus on the social etiquette surrounding the funeral, and gave little thought to the fact that but for him, there would have been no need for a funeral.

Now I asked him straight out: had he driven over his wife with his car? He was insistent that he could remember doing no such thing.

I had learned that the front bumper of his car was damaged, and I asked him if he could explain that. "I don't have any recollection of what happened with the front bumper," he shot back.

I went back to his hazy memory of the moment in which he had killed Bernice. Could he recall the size of the handbag she had hit him with? "It was that large"—he approximated the size with his hand. "Possibly four by six inches."

Suddenly he said, "Sometimes I feel I remember I heard her. I have the feeling I was on the ground when screams called me."

"Why didn't you call the doctor when you knew she was dead?"

"I knew she was dead, but I don't know why I didn't call the doctor."

By this time, I was satisfied that this was not a case of amnesia. He remembered too much for amnesia to have caused the gap in his recollection. It was not that he *could not* recall exactly what had happened; rather, it was more a matter of whether or not he *wanted* the memory. However, it was still not entirely clear whether he was simply a malingerer, or a man whose violent rage had caused him to do something which pained him so greatly that he could not bring himself to remember it.

When I asked him if, in view of the story he had related to me and the police, he should be considered "guilty" of his wife's murder, he replied, "Yes. If you think I killed her, yes, I am guilty." He seemed, if anything, to be avoiding his feelings, which indicated that whatever his mental condition at the time of the murder, he might *now* be in some psychological limbo—neither calm and deliberate nor dissociated, but rather in something approaching a state of panic.

While a defendant's description of and comments on the specifics in a case are useful for getting at his inner thoughts, the general observations that a psychiatrist is able to make from the course of any conversation with a defendant are also extremely important. Van Horn, I realized in time, needed to portray himself as honest and a real gentleman. But he seemed to be trying to convince himself as much as others—as if he were beginning to learn things about himself that were very different from the image he sought to present to himself and to the world.

After several examinations it became clear to me that Van Horn had often been expected to act in ways that were contrary to his nature, that he had often been required to be tolerant and outgoing when in fact he was not. He was a victim of duty; and many of his duties had involved his marriage to Bernice, a difficult person to be with.

This was a man whose conscience told him he should be feeling and doing one thing, when in reality he felt like doing something else. Van Horn had not been raised to express negative feelings, and anger was something he had been trained to avoid. He made it quite clear to me what he thought about friction between people. "Whenever there was an argument," he remarked about his formative years, "I used to walk away."

Van Horn recalled that until his marriage he had wet his bed fairly regularly—an overt sign of immaturity (and, I might add, a habit often found in juvenile delinquents). Even since the marriage, there had been at least a few instances of it. In some fundamental way, it appeared to me, this was an adult who, psychologically, was not fully formed; who had more of the emotional characteristics of the infant and adolescent than one could usually carry successfully into adulthood without having to pay a steep price.

Van Horn complained about having dizzy spells while in custody and made a point of describing similar incidents—including fainting—dating back to his adolescence. They happened ten or twelve times a year, he told me. (He also described several head injuries he had sustained while playing football.) The defense would make much of the dizzy spells at the trial, implying that they manifested the epilepsy shown even more dramatically by his sister—of this I was sure. But his dizzy spells could just as easily be psychologically based, a product of his extreme passive dependency and the concurrent anxiety such feelings engender.

It had taken a good deal of examination to get a firm

handle on what was, in some respects, a complicated situation. But after intense questioning over a period of days, I was able to make my report to the court.

Robert Jett Van Horn had married out of passive acquiescence to Bernice's demands, rather than because he had any great love for her. Once they were married, it appears that the most significant way she satisfied his needs was by helping elevate his social standing. To be prominent in Baltimore's wealthy community, a member of clubs that admitted only the *best* people, it had been necessary for Van Horn to have a well-connected wife. In that sense, she had been more commodity than mate.

Van Horn, during his two-and-a-half-year marriage, had lived with a woman who had many of her own problems, some of them hysterical. His own way of coping with trauma, strengthened over many years, was to draw closer to his own family, especially his mother. He had become increasingly unhappy with his marriage and developed massive resentment and hostility toward his wife, which he had simply not known how to express adequately.

The arguments leading to the fatal event and the murder were the harvest of years of accumulated bitterness. Passive-dependent, fired by pent-up rage, Van Horn had been primed for violence. As it happened, Bernice had set it off with her handbag.

As for his story about beating her to death with his fists, that too was in doubt. Bernice had sustained thirty-two bone fractures and had massive thoracic hemorrhages due to the crushing of her chest. Her body exhibited numerous lacerations and contusions, and her spine had been severed. Moreover, the autopsy photographs showed definite tire marks on her breasts and torso. He might have beaten her, but he had *certainly* run over her with a car.

Van Horn's answers to my questions had been generally coherent. Although somewhat defensive, he seemed, for the most part, to be trying to cooperate. He was well oriented and alert, and his memory was fine—except for the time of the killing. That memory lapse could be any combination of elements—part repression, part effort not to tell me things that could damage him at his trial, for example. But he did not manifest any hallucinations, paranoid or morbid ideas, delusions or, at least presently, suicidal thoughts. He was a bright man who was clearly able to differentiate between right and wrong. Most important, at the time of the crime he had known the nature and quality of his act and fully realized that he had done something wrong. His anxiety notwithstanding, he did not appear to have been criminally insane when he killed his wife, and under the law, he should be held responsible for his crime.

John Grayson Turnbull opted for trial by a panel of judges rather than by a jury. He felt that jurors, as lay people, might not understand—or appreciate—the involved psychological theory that would be used in defending Van Horn from conviction of murder in the first degree. Then too, since Van Horn came from the upper crust of society, the average juror might harbor some class prejudice against him.

The presiding judge, John B. Gontrum, came from an old Baltimore family. Judge Lester L. Barnett was a Republican, like Gontrum, and could be expected to be at least somewhat favorably disposed toward a representative of the city's "better" class of people. The third judge, Michael P. Smith, was a Democrat.

In his opening remarks, Turnbull skillfully and convincingly presented the case for insanity, and succeeded in turning the tables on the prosecution. The judges ruled that the prosecution would have to prove beyond a reasonable doubt that the defendant had been *sane* when the crime occurred. The ruling was a significant victory for the defense, for it placed a double burden of proof on the prosecution: although a defendant is always presumed innocent until proved guilty, he is usually presumed sane until proved insane. This varies from place to place, depending upon state law and, in cases such as this, upon judicial discretion.

Newell was disturbed by the decision, sensing that it might foreshadow more unfavorable rulings to come and, ultimately, the judges' predisposition to look with favor on the defense's case when it came time to hand down a verdict. It certainly would not make things easier for me.

Turnbull was going to try to keep out of the proceedings—or at least minimize—as many elements about the homicide itself as possible. His task was to wrap the case in a kind of psychological mystique—implying, suggesting, conjuring up a mental state for Van Horn beset by misperception, confusion and dissociation. The prosecution, on the other hand, would be bent on illuminating all the specifics that Turnbull would be attempting to sweep under the rug. In the end, our side had the advantage: we had evidence.

The Van Horn family history of "epilepsy" and Robert's own record of fainting spells played a major role in Turnbull's strategy. Dr. Houston Merritt, a noted neurologist, gave a deposition attesting to the fact that Van Horn had epilepsy. Turnbull even managed to find Van Horn's athletic coach from the 1920s, now ninety years old, who testified about one of the defendant's fainting spells.

The defense's main witness, Dr. Manfred Guttmacher, stated that in his expert opinion, Van Horn suffered from schizophrenia, had not known what he was doing when he killed Bernice and therefore should be adjudged innocent by reason of insanity. He further contended that in addition to being schizophrenic, Van Horn was also epileptic—a diagnosis the defense needed to explain the defendant's rage and loss of memory. I was startled that he would make such a claim, since in fact the two conditions almost never occur together; when epileptic seizures continue over a very long period of time, their disorienting effect can bring on a psychosis. But Van Horn had no such history.

The use of expert medical testimony in court is, in some ways, a strange phenomenon. Each side tries to be scientific, but it is evident to the public, especially when experts disagree, just how subjective their professional opinions can be. This doesn't mean that we should do away with the whole idea of seeking testimony from expert witnesses; but it does suggest the need for a critical attitude toward all such testimony. It is useful and believable only if consistent with the facts—physical evidence; the testimony of witnesses; the statements, behavior and personal history of the defendant. Also, there is the irreducible fact that expert witnesses are employed by one side or the other and not brought into a case by some benevolent and neutral third party. No professional worthy of the title "sells" his services, but it is only human to identify, at least somewhat, with the side you're on.

The other doctors speaking for the defense presented

the situation pretty much along the same lines as Dr. Gutt-macher, and I began to think that Turnbull might have overplayed his hand. Increasingly, it seemed to me, the defense would have been better off simply claiming that Van Horn had been emotionally disturbed, extremely dis-traught, not quite himself at the time of the crime, rather than trying to show that he had been literally insane.

Turnbull concluded his presentation with character witnesses who left the court with the impression that this meek, sociable, rather nice fellow and the monster who had beaten his wife to death could be one and the same only if he had been insane. The skillful attorney finished by pointing out that while Bernice was wealthy, Van Horn had plenty of his own money, and therefore *that* could be ruled out as a possible motive (It would have suggested a crime committed out of calculation more than lunacy).

Newell then proceeded to pick apart the elaborately constructed case for the defense. Several psychiatrists were called to refute the diagnosis of schizophrenia. Then Dr. Wechsler testified on the subject of epilepsy. He quite simply—and devastatingly, for the defense—pointed out that the kind of epilepsy being claimed for Van Horn was not consistent with his behavior immediately after the killing. The type in question, an epileptic furor in which the person would act berserk, could not be recovered from quickly enough to have permitted Van Horn to behave with such rationality immediately following the crime.

On the stand, I discussed my findings about the de-fendant, and as I had done in my report, I pointed to Van Horn's longtime resentment and hostility toward his wife as the cause of the murder. He had simply had enough of her. She seriously interfered with his life; he couldn't stand it any longer. Being hit with her handbag was the ultimate indignity, and he had finally lost control of the temper he had so carefully held back for so long.

I emphasized his behavior immediately following the death of Bernice as inconsistent with any part of the diagnosis put forth by the defense. I mentioned Van Horn's brief conversation with Mr. Straw, the farmer; the defendant's care in washing himself and his disposal of his bloodied clothes in the river as acts indicative of a clear state of mind. That he knew his wife was dead also showed that he was conscious and alert. The amnesia after the fact, when he was already in custody, to whatever extent it was authentic, was easily attributed to his pain and fear stemming from the full realization of what he had done. I concluded by stating that in my opinion, Robert Jett Van Horn had been sane when he murdered his wife.

On cross-examination, Turnbull went back to Van Horn's alleged amnesia and epilepsy. The crucial element here was the exact nature of the sister's illness, since Van Horn's affliction was supposed to have been inherited. But the prosecution had done its homework. The sister's hospital records told the tale. For one thing, her electroencephalogram had been negative—highly unusual for someone who supposedly had been suffering from epilepsy for twenty-two years. And even those doctors who still thought she might have had the illness had diagnosed it as a type that is not hereditary.

In fact, a retrospective look at her case indicated that it was highly unlikely that she had had any form of epilepsy. "She was an alcoholic," I reminded Turnbull, and I told him that if he wanted "more information about the condition of Mr. Van Horn's sister, I shall be glad to give it." We had learned that Van Horn's sister had also been a drug addict. Her aging parents, who had known nothing about this, were in the courtroom, and in deference to them and knowing his client could not be served, Turnbull dropped that line of questioning.

In his summary, Turnbull focused on Van Horn's alleged amnesia. The memory gap was authentic. The whole affair was simply a blank in the defendant's mind. The murder was foreign to his client's personality and character, Turnbull proclaimed. "We ask for justice," he dramatically concluded, "for justice in itself is mercy."

But justice is also justice. Newell reiterated the prosecution's case, emphasizing that epilepsy as a cause of the fatal beating had been ruled out. Moreover, he reminded the court, the autopsy report made it clear that Van Horn had run over his wife with an automobile. Nothing in the case indicated that schizophrenia had had anything to do with the crime.

The judges deliberated three hours before concluding that Van Horn had been legally sane at the time of the incident, but that he did in fact suffer from psychological disturbance and that the crime had been committed in the heat of passion.

Van Horn was found guilty of manslaughter and sentenced to ten years in the Maryland penitentiary. He received the sentence with little display of emotion, as if he had expected it (and perhaps thought he deserved it). As he was taken from the courtroom, disappearing through the door that led to the jail, the cream of Baltimore society looked on quietly.

5
CAN FORTY
PSYCHIATRISTS
BE WRONG?

On a chill January morning in 1972, a 707 jet aircraft, TWA Flight 2, was cruising at 39,000 feet over the plains of Iowa, en route from Los Angeles to Kennedy Airport in New York. The time was 4:45 A.M., and there was little sound from the ninety-four passengers and crew of seven. On this cold winter dawn, no one aboard knew or had reason to care about a fellow passenger named Gary Trapnell; nor had anyone any reason to suspect that a hijacking would turn this flight into a living nightmare.

Connie Tokarsky and Diana Pierce, two of the flight attendants, were in the lounge of the first-class section when a passenger approached them. A man of medium height and weight, he had brown hair and eyes, and wore a brown leather car coat with tan trousers. A little earlier, Tokarsky had noticed this passenger because he had been wearing a cast that covered his left arm. The cast was now gone, and his arm was bleeding. He sat down next to

Tokarsky and handed her a note written on a TWA envelope. When he opened his jacket, she saw that he had a handgun tucked under his belt, partially concealed by the outer garment. She read the note:

> YOU ARE NOW BEING HIJACKED
> ACT NATURAL AND LEAD THE WAY TO
> THE CABIN PHONE
> I HAVE A PISTOL AND THERE'S A
> BOMB IN THE AIRCRAFT!

She looked up quickly into his determined eyes and knew he meant it. He ordered her to lead him to the cockpit; there, once inside, he drew the gun, pointed it at one of the three members of the flight crew and ordered: "Put your hands up and don't reach for any guns." To the pilot, Captain Raymond J. Schriber, he gave another order: "Put this plane on autopilot"—which the captain had already done.

"How long can we stay in the air?" he wanted to know. "Plenty of time," he was told. Moving confidently in the crowded cockpit, he coolly instructed the pilot to put him in communication with the ground, and announced to the Chicago Communications Center that TWA Flight 2 had been hijacked—a fact they already knew because the radio microphone had been left open. In return for the release of his 101 hostages, he told them, he wanted $306,800, amnesty and passage to political asylum in Spain, Sweden, France or England. He also asked to talk with President Nixon. Still calm, he ordered the captain to put him in radio communication with his lawyer, Nathan Barone, in Miami, and with a Dallas psychiatrist, Dr.

David Hubbard. Almost as an afterthought, he demanded that black activist Angela Davis be released from the San Jose, California, county jail, and that his friend and one-time accomplice George Padilla be released from prison in Dallas.

The man assured everyone that he was not playing games, and announced that he had concealed a time bomb, with a seven-hour fuse, in the tail section of the plane. He assured the crew members that if they cooperated, no one would be hurt. Captain Schriber promised to take him wherever he wanted to go.

Apparently enthralled with what he was doing, and hungry for attention, the skyjacker sat holding his gun aimed point-blank at the flight crew while he bragged that he had robbed twelve banks in Canada, and told how cleverly he had concealed his weapon in the plaster cast when he boarded the flight in Los Angeles. Once the plane was in the air, he had gone into the lavatory to cut the cast away, accidentally slashing his arm as he did so.

He identified himself as Garrett Brock Trapnell; his nickname was Gary. Captain Schriber began to call him that freely, not realizing that his captor had disclosed his identity quite purposefully. Trapnell knew the FBI was aware of his criminal record, and believed that knowing who he was would lend credence to his threats.

By the time the plane approached the East Coast, fuel was beginning to run low. Trapnell insisted he talk to his lawyer at once. Didn't anybody understand that this was an emergency? he asked, almost plaintively. Giving the pilot instructions for landing at Kennedy, since the fuel was so nearly gone, he ordered Schriber to taxi the plane to a remote corner of the field.

Then he issued a rapid series of commands: "I want this plane fueled. I want the trucks to approach from the front. Nobody leaves the aircraft. If the FBI thinks they're gonna use sharpshooters on me, you're gonna lose some crew members." After every command, he added, "Do you understand that?"

As the plane approached Kennedy Airport, Trapnell began to talk with TWA officials in New York. His chief radio contact was to be Captain James E. Frankum, a vice-president of the airline, who happened to be at the airport that morning.

Trapnell demanded that a corporate jet be sent to Miami to pick up his lawyer, Barone, who had now been located. On the radio, he told Barone: "The FBI can pull the file. I want the money. I want a signed pardon from the President. I want a country in Europe that will accept me as an exile. Now, I'm not kidding. We're gonna refuel at Kennedy, and we're gonna go back in the air. Now, if they try to double-cross me, or play a game with me, ninety-four people aren't going to see tomorrow night. Make arrangements. I don't care who you make it with, but I want my $306,800 back."

New York was nearly in sight by this time. When the plane landed, Trapnell warned, no one was to leave. The instrument panel would tell him if the doors were opened, and he would monitor all ground communications with the aircraft. Nobody was to approach during the refueling. And he now had a new demand: Charles Tillinghast, president of TWA, must call President Nixon personally and tell him that he, Trapnell, wanted to talk to him. Also, he wanted to know, had anyone been able to reach his friend Padilla in the Dallas jail? He claimed that he desperately needed the man's help to control the plane and crew if they went overseas.

Hearing that, Captain Frankum observed cautiously that if Trapnell was planning to go overseas, he would need a new plane and a relief crew.

This made Trapnell angry. "You didn't listen to me!" he shouted. "I want a signed pardon—a signed clemency from the President of the United States. If that's handed to my attorney, I don't need your plane to Europe."

The situation was becoming more dangerous by the minute. Captain Schriber told Trapnell that he had enough fuel for only another hour of flying time, and speaking to the TWA ground officials, he added, "This man is serious. Do whatever you can." Then he tried to soothe Trapnell.

"We'll fly Barone to New York," he said, "and I'll keep communications open to him at all times."

Obviously, Barone was a key figure in Trapnell's getaway plans. The lawyer would be able to ensure that the amnesty and the political documents were genuine, and Trapnell expected him to collect the ransom money while the plane was still in the air.

At that point, Frankum broke in to urge Trapnell to let the passengers go when the plane landed, since they would be of no further use, and after considerable urging from both flight deck and ground, he agreed.

Once the plane was on the ground, Trapnell became anxious. "I want my money *now*," he warned. "I want my money delivered to the plane"—and then, in a bizarre touch of humor: "Let me ask you something. Is that tax-deductible?" He had let the passengers go, but none of his demands had been met and the money had yet to appear.

At 10:30 A.M., with the plane refueled, he gave instructions to take off and fly in a holding pattern over the airport. With the plane at 35,000 feet, he announced to the ground: "I'm sick of this runaround. Either you do what I tell you or I'm going to dive this plane into the terminal." But privately he told the crew, "Hey, fellas, I'm not really going to do it. I'm just telling them that to shake them up so they'll get moving."

Now Dr. David Hubbard, the Dallas psychiatrist, came on the radio to say that he had Padilla in his office, ready to talk to Trapnell. Speaking first in Spanish, then in English, Padilla agreed to take a plane to New York. That seemed to cheer up Trapnell. He was not only calm and perceptive again, he was even gallant. To the four women flight attendants huddled together in the first-class cabin, he said, "I apologize for making you miss your buses and your boyfriends."

He then turned his attention back to Frankum on the ground, and announced that Spain was to be his destination. He wanted the plane ready to take off within four hours. Impossible, he was told. No big jet could be prepared for such a flight in so little time.

With that, Trapnell ordered the plane back to the ground. It landed at 11:30 A.M., taxiing to another remote area of the airport. Belligerent once more, Trapnell demanded to be flown to Dallas to get Padilla.

If he planned to go to Dallas, he was advised, he would need a relief crew, because this one had been on duty since 2 A.M. Trapnell agreed, but he warned that they would have to board the plane exactly as he instructed. The relief crew must have only four members, including a flight attendant. They were to board in shirt sleeves, leaving

98

their jackets behind in the ground transportation that brought them, and this vehicle was not to come nearer than fifty feet to the plane.

These conditions were agreed to. From his vantage point, Trapnell watched the panel truck carrying the new crew approach the plane. They were in shirt sleeves, as he had instructed, and everything seemed to be going as he had demanded. The truck approached the craft and stopped at the prescribed distance, and the new crew emerged from it. Nervously, Trapnell positioned himself just outside the flight deck with the door shielding his body. He ordered Connie Tokarsky to stand in the doorway facing the first-class cabin, with her back to him, so that she would shield him from the new crew as they boarded the plane. The time was 12:30 P.M.

The first of the new crew entered the plane and was frisked by Tokarsky and the first officer of the old crew. Then a second crew member came aboard and was searched. Then came a third man, Gene Frey—an FBI agent. Trapnell seemed to sense that something might be wrong. While Frey was being examined for weapons, the skyjacker came out from behind the door and pushed his gun into the agent's face.

"Are you carrying a gun?" he demanded.

"No," Frey said. It was a lie. He had one concealed in his left boot.

Now the fourth member, James Nelson—also an FBI agent—boarded the plane. He had a captain's flight jacket slung over his arm; there was a gun in one of the pockets. He was also carrying a flight engineer's tool bag. Trapnell, suspicious again, wanted to know what this captain was doing with the bag. At that point, Nelson suddenly pulled

99

the gun from the pocket and fired three shots at Trapnell. Two of the bullets hit him, one in the shoulder and the other in the arm, knocking the revolver out of his hand. Frey jumped Trapnell and subdued him as the hijacker screamed, "I'm shot, I'm shot!"

Ten hours before, Trapnell had come aboard the aircraft with his left arm in a cast. Now he left the plane, lying flat on a stretcher, with his right arm in a sling.

I met Gary Trapnell eight months after his arrest. Peter Schlam, an assistant U.S. attorney in New York, called to ask if I had time to examine him. Like everyone else who had been glued to the radio that day, I knew all about Trapnell and his notorious feat. I was fascinated, and I told Peter to come and see me.

He arrived in my office, a few days later, carrying an overstuffed briefcase. "Garrett Trapnell claims he was insane when he took over the airplane," Schlam told me. "I have all the documents pertinent to this case, and his previous involvements with the law. His record goes back several years."

Emptying the briefcase as he talked, Schlam went on: "He has a long record of bank robberies and holdups, and he's passed hundreds of bad checks. He's been AWOL from the Army, escaped from at least three mental hospitals and made several suicide attempts. Several psychiatrists have declared him insane."

While Schlam watched, I began to flip through pages of hospital, psychiatric, jail, FBI, prison and court records. Almost anything could be found in Trapnell's record— incompetent to stand trial; schizophrenic; schizophrenia with paranoid components; paranoid characteristics; delusional and suicidal. The list went on endlessly. Psychiatrist after psychiatrist had certified his incompetence

100

to stand trial, his unfitness to serve a prison sentence. As I read, my interest in this man intensified, and I looked forward to examining all these documents.

That weekend I studied Trapnell's record. Going through his seemingly bottomless file, I concluded that this man had probably been in more bizarre entanglements with the law and with mental-health professionals than anyone I had ever examined. Also, the reports seemed contradictory. In one, he would appear as cooperative and intelligent, but in the next he would be seen as aggressive, lacking insight, narcissistically concerned with himself. I began to suspect he might be adept at accommodating his reactions to the examiner's attitude.

On a bright October morning I arranged a meeting with Trapnell in New York's Federal House of Detention. I met a tall, slim, good-looking man in his early thirties, dressed in brown trousers and jacket, his shirt open at the collar. He regarded me intently; I had the feeling he was someone who was keenly alert and perceptive, a person to be wary of.

Returning his intent gaze, I noted Trapnell's brown mustache and his dark blond hair combed neatly to one side. On his left hand he wore a big ring, and on the right there was a round scar near the thumb. He was calm enough, but I sensed an underlying tension, which increased visibly when I introduced myself as a psychiatrist for the prosecution. He knew that when he came to trial, some or all of the information I gathered there could be used against him. While he was free to answer my questions, he was. also free to remain silent if he chose. He seemed to have no objection to my taking notes during the interview.

Trapnell understood the charges against him, and it was

also plain after a few minutes that he understood what I was saying to him. But it wasn't apparent just yet how he would respond. Every person I examine responds differently in such circumstances, and the response is usually determined by whether the defense or the prosecution has engaged me. Some prisoners see me at once as an antagonist, someone they must throw off guard, and fool if possible. Others think of me as the man who will keep them out of prison; while the rest simply keep me at bay.

When I interview a defendant, I ask him first about his life, his personal experiences, his childhood, his family background. I try to put him at ease, and at the same time obtain from him some background information relating to his arrest. With Trapnell, however, the interview didn't begin that way. Taking over the conversation himself, he began to elaborate on the skyjacking before we had barely begun. He had nothing to hide, he told me, nothing at all; he didn't remember anything about taking the airplane. I saw that he meant to go on the offensive immediately, and so I asked him to tell me his first memory of the flight.

"I remember being shot," he said in a strong, masculine voice.

"Anything else?"

"No."

Trapnell said he could recall nothing of the flight itself, nor could he remember what he had done on the West Coast, or where he had lived when he was there, although all this was part of his immediate past. It had taken place less than twelve months before.

I found this total lack of memory very strange. Even in schizophrenic psychosis, such complete amnesia is extremely rare. It was incredible to me that Trapnell had suffered a total loss of memory. We had been talking no more than fifteen minutes, and he appeared intent on having me think him mentally ill. I thought it was surprising that in spite of his poor memory, he appeared quite alert, paying attention to every question I asked him, thinking through his answers carefully.

I remembered reading in the newspaper that at his arraignment Trapnell had said, "I'm the one who committed the crime. Everyone knows I'm the one who did it."

Questions were raised in my mind. Did his admission of guilt mean that at some level he wanted to be punished? Did he feel he deserved it for having been caught? Or had he, perhaps, undertaken such a brash and visible crime in the unconscious hope that he *would* be caught? And yet he seemed to think he was too smart to get caught. If that was true, might it not also be possible that he had committed many crimes for which he had never been caught or served time in prison?

But at this point in our relationship, I was more interested to hear about his early years and his family. I didn't pursue the skyjacking itself for the moment. Briskly, without hesitation, he went through the broad outlines of his life—some of which I already knew, but it was instructive to hear it from him. He told me he had been born on January 31, 1938, in Massachusetts. His mother, who had attended Radcliffe, had been only eighteen years old when she married her thirty-six-year-old husband. She later became an alcoholic, he said, and his parents were divorced when Garrett was four.

He lived with his mother until 1949, and then went with his sister to the Panama Canal Zone, where his father, Walter Scott Kennedy Trapnell, was living with his second wife. The senior Trapnell, an Annapolis graduate, had become a commander in the Navy. Later, however, he had been dishonorably discharged, reportedly for operating a brothel in the Zone, although the Navy refused to verify this.

Aside from his father's dubious record, Garrett Trapnell appeared to have come from a family of brave and skillful men. An uncle, Lieutenant General Thomas A. Trapnell, who had been decorated for heroism after the Bataan death march, was later made commander of the 187th Airborne Combat Team in Korea, and was one of the first U.S. military commanders in Vietnam. Another uncle, Admiral Frederick M. Trapnell, like Garrett's father an Annapolis graduate, had been a noted Navy test pilot, and his son Joseph was a captain with Eastern Air Lines. Joseph and another pilot, oddly enough, had been responsible for overpowering a Cuban refugee who, on September 3, 1971 (five months before Garrett's skyjacking), tried to commandeer a jetliner between Chicago and Miami.

Trapnell described these family members to me with great pride, and I could see that if I allowed him to, he would have liked to talk a great deal more about them. But I wanted to move on. What about his mother and grandmother, when he lived with them? Well, he said, those two women had fought each other fiercely over the mother's heavy drinking; they were always battling and pulling each other's hair.

His father died when he was fourteen. They had been playing cards together one evening when his father suddenly began to vomit. Garrett got him to bed, but was sent off to his own room. Next morning, he and his younger sister went to school, but were called home early and told their father had been taken to the hospital and had died there.

It was a great shock, and he cried over it, Garrett told me. "My father was strict, a disciplinarian. He hated lying and hit me with a strap when I did it. But I liked him."

As we talked, Trapnell produced other disturbing memories of his childhood. When he was six years old, a pearl necklace had disappeared from his mother's bureau, and she told everyone he had taken it. "She said she had beaten and beaten me for stealing the necklace, so everyone blamed me. Then later on she found out I hadn't taken it at all." He spoke angrily, but I had a feeling that he was lying and had in fact been the thief.

There was always turmoil in his mother's household, he said. He slept in a large four-poster bed with his mother until he was six or seven. She drank constantly during the day, and, according to him, on weekends she spent her time with cabdrivers in Boston.

"Is this something you heard?" I inquired. "Or did you see it yourself?"

"Everyone knew it," he answered evasively.

In grade school, he did well with languages, particularly Spanish, which he spoke fluently as an adult. At first he told me he had attended school regularly, but when I questioned him further, he admitted that he had sometimes been a truant.

"Did you graduate from high school?" I asked him.

No answer.

"After my father died, my stepmother threw me out of the house," he volunteered instead.

"Why?"

"I don't know."

According to FBI reports, Trapnell had been charged by the police with stealing a pair of shoes at that time, when he was only fifteen. He was placed on probation. I passed over this incident, however, and asked if he could tell me more about his schooling.

Through the intervention of one of his uncles, he said, he had been admitted to the Miami Military Academy in 1953, but did badly there and went AWOL several times. Again, his statement was at odds with the facts. The report of a psychiatric social worker at Jackson Memorial Hospital in Florida, where he had stayed in 1966, disclosed that he had attended Miami Military for only two days, and even in that short space of time had gone AWOL.

Trapnell denied that he had ever repeated any grades. He also said that he couldn't remember any of his teachers. "Do you have a good memory?" I asked him.

"Yes, I think so."

He went on to talk about his sister. "My stepmother kept my sister after our father died, but about two years later she ran away. She got married when she was seventeen, but her husband deserted her and her two children. She remarried and had some more children, but her second husband died of a heart attack."

I had thought at first that Trapnell and his sister had been close, but that turned out not to be true. When he came into court for the first time on a criminal charge, he had tried to persuade her to testify for him, but she did not appear until she was subpoenaed. In fact, from the time Trapnell left Panama in 1953 until 1971, his sister had seen him only three times, including her appearance in court.

As the interview progressed, Trapnell appeared willing,

even eager, to answer my questions, but I sensed that he was also annoyed with me, and it was only later that I discovered why. I hadn't given him the chance to talk about what was *really* on his mind—his long history of mental instability. When I had to repeat my questions, he became belligerent and anxious. Sometimes he was afraid someone might overhear us; but at other times, he was simply confronted with facts he couldn't avoid. Thus the interview became a subtle duel, in which Trapnell was jockeying for position to control the conversation.

"I lived as a street urchin until the Reverend Baldwin sent me to St. Francis' Boys' Home in Salina, Kansas," he said. "I stayed there until 1955; then I ran away, and when I was seventeen, I joined the Army."

"How did you get along in Kansas?" I asked.

"Just fine. I loved it, and there was no trouble. I was even a hero once when I lost two teeth stopping another boy from stealing a car. And I studied hard. I was one of the first boys from the Home chosen to go to public high school. I even had a horse and went riding."

How did he happen to have a horse? Trapnell couldn't say, but he gave me to understand that he had owned it. The record showed, however, that far from being a hero and having his own horse, he had been a troublemaker at the Home.

"What about your wife?" I inquired, changing the direction of the conversation.

"My wife is twenty-one years old," he said.

"And you're thirty-four?"

"What's wrong with that?" he asked, belligerent again.

"Nothing at all. I was just wondering if age difference is a problem."

107

"I'm not a nightclubber," he said defensively, "and I'm not a partyer. I believe in the family, in being at home, having a family structure, and I happen to be married to a woman who believes the same thing."

Trapnell's words belied the real record. In fact he had been married twice before. His first marriage, in 1964, was to a girl from Germany who bore him a daughter. She had divorced him while he was a patient at Clifton T. Perkins State Hospital in Maryland. And in 1967 he had married Susan, by whom he had two more children. After she divorced him in 1970, Susan's new husband had had to warn him to stay away from her. He had met his current wife, Susanne, while he was a patient at the Pinel Institute in Montreal, from which he had escaped in January 1971.

He was vague about his employment, saying only that he had been working on an airplane.

"When?" I asked.

"A while ago."

"How long ago?"

No answer. Instead, he told me he had reenlisted in the Army in 1957, but he didn't say that he had been given an undesirable discharge. His reenlistment, in fact, had been fraudulent, and he had also stolen government property.

Trapnell's answers grew less and less precise. He was being very careful not to volunteer any information that would tend to incriminate him. More and more, he was on the defensive.

Fortunately, I had his record to fill in the blanks and give me guidance. I knew that later in the year, after he was discharged from the Army, he had committed several bank robberies, with the help of two accomplices. They were all caught, but while the others were convicted and sentenced to prison, Trapnell was declared insane and escaped jail. After another arrest for bank robbery, he claimed auditory and visual hallucinations and was sent to Spring Grove State Hospital in Maryland, where he was diagnosed as having a schizophrenic reaction, chronic paranoid type. Discharged in 1959, he was transferred to the Baltimore County Jail, but was released because of insanity, so the discharge papers said.

Free again on February 28, 1961, Trapnell nevertheless was soon readmitted to the same mental hospital, claiming that he felt irresistibly suicidal, and was having terrifying visual and auditory hallucinations and was certain he would commit more robberies. He also declared the FBI was after him.

The doctors diagnosed him as paranoid, but what they didn't know was that the FBI *was in fact* after him, and he had come back to Spring Grove because it was the safest hideout he could think of, and the only way to avoid prosecution. He openly admitted all this more than two years later, when he was in the Kent County jail in Maryland.

As I read through the dry, official account of Trapnell's incredibly colorful life, I felt amazement, almost bordering on admiration, at this man's ingenuity. Although I had examined many criminals in my time, I had had yet to meet one with his wit and imagination. If only, I thought, those mental resources had been turned toward something constructive: what he might have accomplished!

A month after his readmission to Spring Grove, he escaped. After passing several worthless checks between 1961 and 1963, he was arrested again and committed once more to Jackson Memorial Hospital in Florida, claiming insanity. There he was diagnosed as a psychopath—selfish, lying and antisocial, but not psychotic—and the court, seeming not to know quite what to do with him, sent him to jail. He was soon transferred to Clifton T. Perkins State Hospital, where he was diagnosed as having schizophrenic reactions with paranoid components. Although he was considered competent to stand trial, the verdict was the familiar "Not guilty by reason of insanity."

During the next several years, Trapnell repeated his pattern of criminal behavior followed by insanity pleas. His astonishing arrest record piled up. Bank robbery in Canada. Impersonating a police officer in New Mexico. Passing bad checks in California. Burglary. Theft. In September 1969, making another appearance in court, this time in California, once more he was adjudged not guilty because of insanity and his case was dismissed.

Early in 1970 in California, he had met a topless dancer whom he talked into going to Las Vegas with him. He got her drunk and next day told her they had been married the night before. He told his new "wife" that he had just talked with his mother, who was terribly ill, and he had to leave immediately for Florida. Unfortunately, he had no money, and could he please use her credit cards? Lovingly (and gullibly), she gave them to him, and after a tearful leavetaking, he flew off to Florida, where he chartered an airplane which he piloted himself to the Bahamas. He and an accomplice robbed a jewelry store in Freeport of $100,000 and with the police in hot pursuit, escaped by plane to Florida.

After the robbery in the islands, he pulled off other bank robberies in Montreal, and there, claiming insanity as always, he was admitted to the Pinel Institute, from which he presently escaped. Arrested a little later in Syracuse, he was extradited to Miami, where he was once more found insane, and the extradition to the Bahamas was called off.

While he was in Miami that year, Trapnell had bought a fifty-seven-foot twin-motored luxury yacht for $306,800. I asked him where he had gotten so much money.

"From several bank robberies in Canada," he said, "but don't ask me about them, because I don't remember." (I had to stifle a laugh.)

He did recall that he had acquired $450,000 through the robberies, but he was vague about any other details, informing me that he could only repeat what he had been told by the district attorneys, or had read in their reports or indictments. Later, he changed his story entirely and told me with a perfectly straight face that he had found the money in his mother's closet.

How had he happened to buy the yacht? I asked. Well, that was quite a story too. One day in 1971, while he was staying at a Miami hotel, Trapnell told me, he had found a new, fifty-seven-foot yacht listed for sale in a yachting magazine. It was managed by a man named James Fahey. Trapnell began negotiating with him to buy it for $306,800, and the deal was made. He was supposed to pay by check. But on the day before the official closing, Trapnell called a notary public to the boat and asked him to witness the signing of a bill of sale by Fahey. Later, the notary said that during this transaction, the man who called himself Fahey had not said a word. Next day, Trapnell failed to appear at the closing, and the boat's owner, a man named Kinney, went to look for him. He found Trapnell already aboard the yacht, insisting it was already his and asserting he had paid for it in full.

Was this strange transaction legitimate? James Fahey could have corroborated Trapnell's payment, but unfortunately, he was no longer around. He had vanished mysteriously, and has not been found to this day. Luckily for Kinney, he held a lien on the yacht, and it could not be sold except in his presence. Consequently, his corporation was able to sue successfully, and a marshal seized the craft from Trapnell.

At last we had the explanation for Trapnell's demands for cash after he skyjacked the 707. By some strange reasoning process, he believed the $306,800 he had paid for the yacht had been swindled from him by the United States Government.

I had trouble getting straight answers from Trapnell about his yachting adventure, but when I began to ask about his various hospitalizations, his eyes lit up and he sat straighter in his chair, all eager attention. Clearly, this was what he wanted to talk about, and he began to tell me, almost urgently, about his many stays in mental hospitals. I realized that to Trapnell each one of them represented a success, a triumph, a confirmation of his power.

He told me he had been in Maryland State Hospital twice, although he was evasive about the details. He had also been in a Florida hospital—probably in 1963, but he wasn't sure. When he was in the Army in 1958, he had shot himself in the abdomen and been taken to the hospital unconscious. Later research substantiated this story, but the year was 1956; he was in the hospital for six weeks. There had been several such "suicide" attempts. While he was in Maryland State Hospital in 1956, he had cut

112

his forearm (superficially) in several places, and in June 1957, during his Army service, he cut his left arm (he always avoided his wrists) and was taken to the base hospital at Ford Ord, California, then was transferred the following month to Letterman Army Hospital in San Francisco. When he talked to me about these suicide attempts, I felt that Trapnell was deliberately trying to mislead me. Dramatically, he declared that during one of them, he had seemed to hear his father's voice saying, "You're a disgrace! The only way you can save yourself is to kill yourself."

He continued to try. In 1963, he cut himself again, and then attempted to hang himself in the hospital, but was cut down. After that, he declared, he had stopped hearing the destructive voices urging him on.

Although he described many of his suicidal efforts in minute detail, he appeared completely unaware of the contradiction between his vivid recall of them and the total amnesia he affected about his crimes.

By this time it was becoming clear how the scores of psychiatrists who had preceded me with Trapnell could have been fooled. There aren't many people, sane or insane, willing to go to the lengths Trapnell did to prove to the world that he was not responsible for his criminal actions. Still, the nagging question remained: Why had he made such a sustained and bizarre effort, including the apparent suicide attempts, however doubtful they might be? What, in short, did Trapnell *really* want?

I thought I knew the answers. For one thing, of course, he wanted to avoid responsibility for his crimes. But there did appear to be some fantasies of self-destruction present. The men in his family had been distinguished members of the Armed Forces, and he had once aspired to their success, but as time went on, he had been more and more conscious of his failure in life. "My whole family was excellent—excellent," he told me."I'm the only one who's been in jail." Yet in one endeavor, Trapnell had been enormously successful. He had made his mark as a charlatan. He was a consummate malingerer—and he knew it. From this, if from nothing else in his life, he got ego gratification.

As he talked about his confinements in mental hospitals across the country—in Florida, Maryland, California, Texas and New York—Trapnell repeatedly gave me the diagnoses of the psychiatrists, and they were invariably the same: paranoid schizophrenia. I asked if he'd seen these reports.

"Yes."

"How come?"

"Because they were given to my lawyer."

"Did they become part of the court proceedings?"

Trapnell nodded, and remarked: "It's the government that's raised the question of insanity."

I knew that wasn't the case. His lawyer, Gregory Perrin, had asked that his client be given a psychiatric examination after he had been transferred to the surgical ward of Bellevue Hospital in New York for the removal of the bullets from his arm following the skyjacking. Since he had a history of hospitalization and crimes extending over nearly twenty years, the request was routine. A Bellevue psychiatrist returned the drearily familiar verdict, paranoid schizophrenia, and Trapnell was taken to the prison ward of the psychiatric wing, where he was guarded by three FBI men, since this was a federal crime.

He couldn't remember exactly how many mental hospitals he had been in, Trapnell told me, but he thought it might be as many as ten.

"They all found you had a psychosis?" I inquired.

"Yes. I have a transcript of five sodium amytal [truth serum] sessions at Bellevue. They sent me a transcript." He went on, speaking now with great conviction: "There was a Greg Ross and a Gary Trapnell. It came out as a split. The whole thing was thoroughly and completely explained to me by the doctor. Every single day for a hundred and some days, this doctor spent two hours a day with me, and one sodium amytal session lasted two hours and a half. I went through a psychological meat grinder—if you know the expression—at Bellevue. The doctor explained it all to me. He said there were variances between Greg's father and Gary's father, between Greg's mother and Gary's mother. I've seen the transcripts."

"Who is this Greg?"

"He's supposed to be the other personality. I knew nothing about Greg, or anything else, until the sodium amytal."

Again, Gary's version was far from true. At the trial later on, it was shown that Trapnell had used several aliases, among them "Greg Ross," before the skyjacking. "Greg" was his own invention.

I brought the questioning back to the yacht once more.

"There was a court battle, then, and you lost the boat?"

"Right."

"In 1971?"

"Yes, sir."

"What happened after that?"

"I lost my business [He had leased a marina]...because a newspaper article about the court battle depicted me as a former mental patient, and the people who owned the hotel I'd leased the marina from no longer wanted me around."

Trapnell paused and, switching abruptly back to the present, volunteered that he might get a "suspended life sentence," followed by psychiatric care, "so somebody could help me." That was the first time I had ever heard of a suspended life sentence, but Trapnell went on in a friendly, confiding voice: "The court has been sending me to psychiatrists, and a trial date should be set." Apparently he had no doubt that he would be found insane.

"When you were on the outside, you never sought psychiatric help, did you?" I asked.

"No, I didn't," Trapnell said briefly.

I thought it strange, in view of his long psychiatric history, that he had never voluntarily sought help himself. Plainly, psychiatry had never come into the picture except in the aftermath of a crime.

Our first interview had lasted more than two hours.

II

When I went back for a second examination, Trapnell refused at first to come down from his cell. At last he consented, and when he finally appeared, he was coughing, complaining about his asthma and breathing difficulties. In spite of that, he smoked incessantly.

As we sat down, he cried out, almost like a child, "You don't believe me!" and I understood why he had been slow about coming down. Trapnell was a perceptive man.

Our second interview developed from the first, with the

emphasis on his many stays in the hospitals. At the end of it, he asked me anxiously, "What did you find out about my mental condition?"

"I'm sorry, but I can't answer that question," I said.

At this, he became angry and agitated, *insisting* that I answer. I told him to stop asking because it was too early for me to give an opinion.

In all my years of practice, no defendant had ever asked me this question. Anyone truly suffering from a paranoid schizophrenic condition isn't concerned about what anyone thinks of him. Often he knows about his condition, and if he doesn't he won't ask. Truly paranoid schizophrenic people will try to convince an examiner that they are well, rather than the opposite, as Trapnell was doing. I realized it would be highly gratifying to him if I told him that I'd concluded he had schizophrenia and was ill, because once again he would have succeeded through cunning in achieving his goal.

With that in mind, I saw the case in perspective for the first time. Here was a terribly destructive man who had been carrying on criminal activities for twenty years. His crimes had to be stopped, and my profession had given me the tools to do it. By combining my forensic experience with the insight into his behavior gained from psychiatric expertise, I knew it was possible to halt Gary Trapnell, this time in court. I set down in my report the conclusions I had come to—that Trapnell was sane and that he had counterfeited schizophrenia so cleverly, he had fooled dozens of psychiatrists—and gave it to the prosecutor, complete with the evidence supporting my opinion.

Trapnell went to trial in Federal Court, Eastern District, New York, charged with air piracy, in December 1972.

Pleading not guilty by reason of insanity, he was confident that he would win this court battle as he had all the others. The procedure in such a case is established by law. If a defendant is adjudged fit to stand trial, as Trapnell was, the next question to be asked is this: had the defendant, as a result of mental disease or defect, lacked substantial capacity to know or appreciate the wrongfulness of his conduct, or conform his behavior to the requirements of the law? If the answer is yes, the defendant is then adjudged not guilty by reason of insanity.

Trapnell's lawyers called to the stand the Bellevue psychiatrist who had interviewed the skyjacker after his crime. He testified that Trapnell had compared himself to Napoleon, and that he had asserted that "voices" had told him to do what he was accused of doing. His diagnosis, therefore, was paranoid schizophrenia. Then a staff psychologist at Bellevue testified that he had put Trapnell under sodium amytal in order to explore the possibility of a dual personality.

What were his findings? The doctor testified that he had found there was a primary personality, Garrett Trapnell, but there was a second personality called Gregory Ross. "He had divided not only himself, but also he had divided people who were close to him and had, so to speak, incorporated their characteristics inside himself in order to build his own identity. In other words, Gregory Ross got inside Trapnell and made him do things."

I was amazed to hear this description. Not only was there the matter of his previous use of "Gregory Ross" as a convenient alias, but it seemed clear to me, on the basis of what the defendant had told me in our interviews, that this diagnosis was actually Trapnell's own description of his case.

118

For the prosecution, Assistant U.S. Attorney Schlam called to the stand the convict named Padilla, whose freedom Trapnell had demanded during the skyjacking. Padilla told of meeting the accused in a Florida hospital, where his new friend had taught him how to prove himself crazy through tricks designed to fool the experts. Trapnell had given Padilla a kind of guided tour through the Rorschach and other psychological tests. During a lengthy, and often stormy, cross-examination, Padilla stuck to his story.

Then Schlam produced a surprise witness, a journalist named Cyrus Jacob Berlowitz, who testified that in April 1971, nine months before the skyjacking, he had been assigned by *True* magazine to interview Trapnell, at his request. The result was seventeen hours of taped conversation. *True* had not published the interview, but the tape was entered on the court record. It was played back at the trial, and it confirmed my conclusions about Trapnell.

With remarkable candor, he related that in California he had been told by a lawyer to plead not guilty by reason of temporary insanity, observing that "temporary" precludes hospitalization. "In most states," he said, "they'll find me not guilty and ship you to a goddamned state hospital for a year. But this 'temporary' shot, which is much harder and more intricate, takes a little bit more finesse. Precludes the hospitalization period..."

Trapnell went on to say in the Berlowitz interview that if the journalist printed what he was telling him, "you blow my whole gig.... If that part is ever published, there won't be any reactions, but there will be a hell of a lot of indignant psychiatrists and judges." He cited another lawyer who, he declared, would "tell you that I'm a classic N.G.I. [not guilty by reason of temporary insanity] plea—

119

it's a license to kill....I could go out on the street in New York, shoot ten people, and in six months I'd be free. Isn't that weird?"

How had he first developed this seemingly foolproof technique, this "license to kill"? Trapnell was equally frank about that. On "one of my first busts," he told Berlowitz, "a lawyer came to me and said, 'Trap, look, you are going to prison for twenty years, or you can go to the state hospital.' So I went to the state hospital....I read more goddamned books on psychiatry and psychology than probably any psychology student ever will in any school in the world." And he went on to prove the depth of his knowledge by describing in clinical terms the psychiatric evaluation and diagnosis of paranoid schizophrenia, and of what he called "the classic dual personality, compounded by paranoia, the sense of being persecuted." He even knew that his acquittals would be based on a precedent established in a landmark case of 1843, since known in law as the M'Naghten Rule. He admitted to Berlowitz that he had invented the name "Greg Ross" for the other half of his presumptive split personality, and told why. "...Using the split personality, if Greg Ross commits a crime...and the Greg Ross aspect submerges after he is put in prison, and the Gary Trapnell aspect emerges...then Gary Trapnell is not responsible legally for what Greg Ross does....Ten psychiatrists— put them together and they all come up with a different diagnosis. Or—varying diagnoses. I probably know more about psychiatry...than your average resident psychiatrist—I can bullshit the hell out of one in ten seconds."

At the end of the Berlowitz interview, Trapnell offered an admirable summary of his life of crime, and how he had avoided paying for it. "The fact remains," He said, "that I have committed all of these crimes and have never gotten a number for any of them. And it's like—it's your system, baby; it's not mine....It's the fallacy of your legal system.

"You see," he went on, "here we get back to prosecution—it's either black or white; there's no gray matter. Either the man falls under this antiquated psychiatric scheme of things, or he doesn't; a guy can be the most honest guy in the world and have a mental quirk, and go to prison, whereas a guy who can bullshit himself into a situation gets cut loose. I have no right to be on the streets today. That's the way I feel about it....I am being very brutal with myself...and the only reason I am free today is because of the system we have devised."

I sat back listening to this tape with considerable satisfaction. Here was Trapnell condemning himself in his own words. I could understand even better now his anxiety at our last interview, when it was becoming clear to him that he had encountered a psychiatrist whom he could not "bullshit."

My own testimony on the witness stand was almost anticlimactic. I testified, in substance, that Trapnell had learned how to fool a long list of psychiatrists by mimicking the symptoms of insanity. He had also been successful in deceiving judges, district attorneys, correctional and probation officers, persuading them all to believe that he was insane. Moreover, having read a great many books on psychiatry and psychology, he was able to figure out and explain all the symptoms he claimed to have. Nevertheless, he had inadvertently convinced me that he wasn't insane. "Trapnell is a very perceptive man," I told the court, "and also quite seductive."

I described how I had come to my conclusion. My first

121

suspicion of Trapnell's "insanity" arose because of the ease with which he had talked about his symptoms. Whatever we might be discussing, he always returned to the subject of his mental state. When I had asked him about his crimes, he talked about them, cautiously and defensively, but he was eager to manipulate the interview back to his alleged mental illness.

As for the split personality, the incidence of true double personality is very rare, in spite of the common impression to the contrary inspired by several well-publicized cases. I may have seen one case in forty years. In the entire literature, only twenty people in the last twenty-five years have been identified as having multiple personalities. Even some of these cases are of doubtful authenticity, because the plurality of personalities may have involved role-playing.

I described the care with which Trapnell had planned the air piracy: making a cast to conceal the gun; writing the skyjack note; demanding a presidential pardon (a clear indication that he felt guilty); cutting off the cast to get to the gun; threatening the crew with it—all these were conscious, well-planned, manipulative actions. In accordance with New York State law on insanity, at the time of the skyjacking Garrett Trapnell did not lack substantial capacity as a result of mental disease or defect to appreciate the wrongfulness of his behavior or to conform his behavior to the requirements of the law.

During his lengthy cross-examination, the defense attorney suggested that the demands for the freedom of Angela Davis, and some of his other requests, were not consistent with a well-calculated criminal venture. It was true, I agreed, that there were certain aspects of the skyjacking, like these, which showed Trapnell trying to draw attention to himself; but as I told the court, "Bravado in itself is not a symptom of paranoid schizophrenia." If that diagnosis were true, I went on, and if this were a man mentally incapacitated by hallucinations, delusions, confusion and feelings of persecution, he could not have carried out the crime. Using a cast to conceal the weapon, and writing the note, were inconsistent with such an illness. "Schizophrenia is not a headache," I concluded. "It is a very serious condition that you cannot walk in and out of."

After five weeks of trial, the case went to the jury. Almost from the moment they retired, eleven jurors were for convicting Trapnell, and one, a psychiatric social worker, favored acquittal because of insanity. After several days, the jury announced itself deadlocked, and when the deadlock showed no sign of being broken, the judge declared a mistrial. Trapnell was returned to jail until a new trial, which was set for May 7, 1973.

At the second and much shorter trial, during which I again testified, the jury took only three hours to find Trapnell guilty. It marked the end of an extremely difficult piece of detective work for me, and the close of a criminal career for him.

Hidden beneath the tremendous mass of psychiatric and criminal records there had been lurking a mentality capable of blocking everyone's efforts to perceive it. When Trapnell was finally revealed to be a dangerous criminal with an extraordinary talent for malingering, his cries of protest were loud, but this time there was no way out. He was given a life sentence.

Some questions remained. For one, how had Trapnell

been able to fool so many psychiatrists? In retrospect, given the background of his far-ranging activities—at least twenty serious crimes, innumerable arrests, scores of jails, dozens of mental institutions, three suicide attempts—it would have been very easy to believe him insane. The sheer abundance of his aberrant behavior supported such a diagnosis.

His road to deception could be traced. It appeared likely that he had begun slowly and quietly to misrepresent his state of mind, saying that he was depressed, that he heard voices or that he was afraid he might kill someone. Then, little by little, he had developed these notions more deliberately, especially after he discovered how simple it was to avoid imprisonment by doing so. A perceptive and observant man, he paid careful attention to the doctors' questions; he learned more and more about his "mental illness" from every examination he was given.

His examiners did not realize it, but they were giving him a postgraduate course in how to appear to be out of his mind.

In the end, he could speak with ease about all the symptoms the doctors mentioned—hallucinations, delusions, depressions, sleeplessness, murderous and suicidal impulses. All these phenomena came to form a significant part of Trapnell's "schizophrenic" pattern of symptoms. I also suspected that the psychiatrists who examined him later were influenced by the diagnoses made earlier by their colleagues. Add to all this a final and formidable factor: the access he had gained, through his lawyers, to his own psychiatric reports—something any psychiatrist should have objected to strenuously.

Working carefully over a period of seventeen years,

Trapnell had been able to build up his syndrome of symptoms so that they appeared clinically genuine. When one adds his seductive personality and his talent for deception and manipulation, it's easy to understand why most psychiatrists were convinced of his illness.

But there was another question not quite so easy to answer. How could a man as intelligent as Trapnell have become a criminal? As a product of a broken home, he had had neither stable male nor female adults in his immediate family with whom he could identify. His alcoholic mother was overly possessive, yet incapable of nurturing. He was probably looking for a genuinely protective mother, as he made clear to me in a dream he related during our talks. "A man is shooting at me," he said, "and a woman jumps between us and gets shot. Then I wake up," He had no associations to this dream himself.

Trapnell's father died when he was fourteen, and after that he had to shift for himself. After his upbringing in a family where brutality was the norm, it was brutality that became his guide. He developed an aimless life pattern, filled with deception and violence, meanwhile competing to become a person he could never be, to live up to his family's military tradition. Narcissistic, exhibitionistic, unable to find a real self, he learned to play a role by means of a shortcut—crime. He discovered how to manipulate people, how to take advantage of anyone for his own gratification.

Trapnell was a psychopath, a man with some strange and antisocial character traits. But he was not insane; not—to use the medical term—psychotic. He suffered from a severe character disorder, but was not disabled by mental illness as the psychotic is. He *knew* what he was doing and had the ability to control his behavior.

About two years after Trapnell was sentenced, I went down to the lockup in the Federal Courthouse on Foley Square in New York to examine another prisoner. Standing alone in the dark and echoing corridor, the iron-barred cell doors stretching away ahead of me on both sides, I heard a voice suddenly call out, "Dr. Abrahamsen, I'll get you!" The voice was familiar. I turned around and began making my way back the length of the corridor, peering into each cell as I passed. At one of them, I stopped and stood quietly. Slowly, a figure emerged from the dark shadows of the cell. It was Trapnell. He looked at me silently, and I returned his gaze. Neither of us said a word.

6
UNMASKING
SON OF SAM

A bizarre series of nighttime murders in New York City shocked and fascinated the country in 1976 and early 1977. For an interminable year, millions of New Yorkers became nighttime hostages as the killer—whose trademark was his weapon, a .44-caliber revolver—stalked his victims, usually young women sitting with their dates in parked cars. In cryptic notes to the police and the media, he referred to himself as the "Son of Sam."

The agony ended on August 10, 1977, with the arrest of a young man named David Berkowitz. He had, according to the police, set a grisly record. He had shot and killed five young women and a young man, and his reign of terror had been the longest by a single murderer in the city's history.

People were stunned by the first published photographs of Berkowitz. They saw a face that was soft, round and feminine; he had a sweet, almost seductive smile. He appeared to be mild and gentle, a nice Jewish boy from the Bronx, every mother's son. Was this the brutal killer whose activities had been reported in newspapers ranging from the Vatican's *L'Osservatore Romano* to *Izvestia*?

Berkowitz readily confessed. He had committed the crimes at the behest of demoniacal "voices"—which he heard through the barking of dogs, especially from one owned by a six-thousand-year-old man named "Sam"— whose demands he was helpless to resist. The apparently random killings had created so much fear and tension that most people, needing some explanation for such gruesome and otherwise incomprehensible acts, were ready to be persuaded that he was sincere in what he said.

The criminal-justice system, of course, was less easily persuaded. One of the most notorious mass murderers in history was now in custody. He had confessed. What was to be done with him? It was understood that he would be locked up somewhere, since in New York State the death penalty applies only to prisoners who commit murder while already serving a life sentence. But the question was where he should be confined, under what circumstances and for how long. Could he be held accountable for what he had done? How would the system define and judge his crimes?

Should the case get as far as a trial, it was a foregone conclusion that he would be found guilty. But the man seemed to be out of his mind, and the outcome of the case would actually hinge on the result of a competency hearing, a judicial procedure that would determine whether he was mentally capable of being tried. If he was found to be incompetent, he would be placed in a psychiatric institution, to remain there until he was adjudged sufficiently sane to go to trial.

A single judge, aided by consulting psychiatrists, would

determine Berkowitz' competence. His decision would depend on the answers to several questions: Could Berkowitz recall the details of his crimes? Did he know who he was and where he was? Did he understand the charges against him? Could he stand the stress of a trial; and equally important, was he capable of cooperating with his lawyers in his own defense? Under the law, the defendant could be emotionally ill and yet capable of standing trial.

Sixteen days after Berkowitz' arrest, I found myself sitting in a small, dingy yellow cubicle on the prison ward of the Kings County Hospital. Brooklyn District Attorney Eugene Gold had engaged me to examine Berkowitz for the prosecution.

Face-to-face conversations with killers were nothing new to me, and although I did not meet a mass murderer every day, I was familiar enough with the relevant cases—the Charlie Starkweathers, Richard Specks, Charles Mansons and their kind—to have a sense of what I might expect to find. Still, what happened next was unsettling.

I had been told that there would be a delay before I could see the prisoner because the corridors had to be cleared. In my many years as a forensic psychiatrist, I had never witnessed such a degree of security. Everyone seemed to be afraid of him; the authorities also feared that he might be attacked by another prisoner.

As I sat in that grim place at a desk worn by years of use, I suddenly felt a presence. Turning, I saw that a young man had entered silently. He stood there, just inside the door, wearing the prison hospital's faded blue, pajamalike uniform. Outside the door, which had been left slightly ajar, sat a young guard, positioned so that he had a direct view of the prisoner. As Berkowitz loomed over me, a smile played on his lips, and I wondered what secret satisfaction, amusement, perhaps contempt he harbored.

As I got up to introduce myself, he interrupted me and, still smiling, announced in a determined tone:

"I know who you are; you're Dr. Abrahamsen. I read your book *The Murdering Mind.*" He paused. "The book was good."

None of the hundreds of murderers I had examined had ever mentioned reading anything about the psychological side of homicide. Berkowitz had found my book in the Yonkers Public Library and had also read books by other authors about Nathan Leopold and Richard Speck.

"I like to read about murder and murderers," he said. "It's a recent interest of mine, for a little over two years."

His ability to sustain such a concentrated interest hardly suggested the inner confusion usually present in an insane person. Two court-appointed psychiatrists who had already examined him had reported that Berkowitz had developed a rather elaborate paranoid delusional system and had concluded that he was insane and unfit to stand trial. But my initial impression was that he was alert, highly intelligent and perceptive; he spoke easily, often animatedly.

An individual who imagines that he is possessed by demons who have commanded him to kill is insane (the legal term) and psychotic (the medical term). Such a person would be suffering from paranoia—contrary to popular belief, an extremely rare illness—which is marked by distorted beliefs that are impervious to reason; or from schizophrenia, a thought disorder characterized by confusion, loss of memory and an inability to understand what is going on within or around the individual. A schizophrenic could be said to have a disorganized personality and ordinarily could not hold a job.

Berkowitz had been working at the post office on a regular eight-hour shift at the time of his arrest. In the course of my interviews with him, I was to visit the Bronx facility where he had worked and discovered that there was a constant, tremendous volume of noise, which made it difficult to carry on a conversation. I was puzzled, because Berkowitz had told me that he was sensitive to noise.

I talked to several people who had worked with him, and each spoke of his courteous and gentlemanly ways. One woman said: "He even walked us to the car once. We got off at twelve-thirty A.M. My friend was parked on a deserted street a few blocks away, and we were glad to have someone walking us to the car. We were afraid of going there alone because of all of the stories about the Son of Sam."

When Berkowitz discussed his crimes in interviews and letters, it was quite evident that he recalled exactly when and under what circumstances he had committed them.

On July 29, 1976, in the Bronx, he shot and killed Donna Lauria and wounded Jody Valente.

"All of the shootings were between several minutes to an hour, yes. The first was twenty minutes. This time was spent stalking and watching. I walked around the block several times. I checked out alleyways. I looked up to windows of all the apartment buildings to see if anyone was looking out. But I was secretly hoping that they'd drive away."

The second shooting, in Flushing, Queens, occurred on October 23, 1976, when Carl DeNaro and Rosemarie Keg-

DAVID ABRAHAMSEN, M.D.

nan were wounded. It took "about ten minutes. I could
have waited longer but I was anxious. I wanted to get it
over with and then head home."

The third time, he killed Donna DeMasi and Joanne
Lomino in Floral Park, Queens, November 27, 1976. He
did this "within five minutes. I saw them on the porch.
I drove my car around the corner and parked it. I then got
out, walked directly to the porch up the street and fired."

In Forest Hills, Queens, January 30, 1977, Berkowitz
shot Christine Freund and John Diel. "I saw them get into
the car and I walked up the street. I walked several hundred
feet, turned around and headed back to the car they were
seated in with the engine running. I aimed and fired. This
took about five minutes." John Diel was wounded and
Christine Freund died.

The fifth shooting took place on March 8, 1977, again
in Forest Hills. The victim was Virginia Voskerichian. "I
walked around for a long time—just walking and thinking. I spotted this girl walking up the street. I raised my
gun and shot her once. This took only seconds. But during
that evening I had passed dozens of potential victims. I
don't know why I chose her. I could hardly make out her
facial features in the darkness. However, I was on the
street for several hours—just walking, thinking and
prowling. Now that I look back at this, none of it makes
any sense."

On April 17, 1977, in the Bronx, Valentina Suriani and
Alexander Esau were shot. "This time I again had been
cruising for hours—about six hours. I was headed up
toward Yonkers along the Hutchinson River Parkway service road when I saw two heads over the seat of the car
as I approached from behind. I then drove my car around

132

the corner and parked. I walked towards the car, dropped a note at the scene, then opened fire."

On June 26, 1977, the seventh shooting took place, again in Queens. The victims were Judy Placido and Salvatore Lupo. "Again, I had been walking and staking out this area for hours. I saw them and just finally decided that I must do it and get it over with. Believe it or not, I had no real desire to keep at this. Yet I did. Both were wounded."

Berkowitz' eighth and last shooting, in which he killed Stacy Moskowitz and almost blinded Robert Violante, took place on July 31, 1977, in Brooklyn. He told me:

"I had come from work at ten-thirty P.M. and stopped at a diner and had a little snack. Left the gun in the car. I don't think I had the rifle in the car. I went out to Queens and Brooklyn and had to look around. There was nobody in Queens. So I moved over to Brooklyn....

"I saw her and her boyfriend making out in the car. Then they left the car, walked over the walk bridge and went along the path by the water.

"After about twenty minutes, they returned to the car, made out some more and then came to where I was by the swings. I watched Stacy on the swing and they stopped swinging. Her and her date then started to kiss passionately for several minutes. At this time, I too was sexually aroused. I had an erection.

"Shortly after their deep-kissing they went back to the car. If my memory is correct, they made out a little more and then just sat inside the car talking....

"I walked a hundred feet. Just walked up to it [the car], pulled out the gun and fired into the car on the passenger's side. I fired four bullets."

Berkowitz' mind was clearly not disorganized; in fact,

even by the end of the first interview, it was clear to me that he exhibited none of the symptoms of schizophrenia. Still, there was the possibility that he was a true paranoid, as he had been diagnosed by the two court-appointed doctors. But I doubted that diagnosis too.

My years of work in psychiatric criminology had taught me that the more exceptional, irregular and unnatural a case may seem to be, the less mysterious it often is in the end. In very complicated situations, a thorough examination is the only way to extricate the truth from a confusing mass of detail.

The initial sessions with Berkowitz were not easy going. When I introduced certain subjects—his childhood and family life, primarily—which might yield important information on the nature of his personality, Berkowitz often resisted, drifting away to talk about his demons.

Since David Berkowitz' hallucinations were central to the question of whether or not he was sane enough to stand trial, it was essential to determine whether in fact they were real to him—whether they truly existed in his mind and controlled his actions. I asked him in our initial interview if he could remember the first time the demons had appeared.

"I began to hear them just after I moved to Yonkers," he told me. He had moved from an apartment in the Bronx to New Rochelle in February 1976, and then to Yonkers three months later. But I remembered that he had admitted to having tried to murder a young woman with a knife on Christmas Eve 1975—which meant that he had attempted his first murder without being "commanded" by the demons.

"Who told you to kill?" I inquired, pressing the point.

"Sam Carr." Sam Carr actually lived near Berkowitz, and he owned a dog.

"Where did you get the idea about him?"

"A long story," he answered curtly. For the first time he appeared flustered and began to fidget. The bravado he had displayed in answering my previous questions abruptly disappeared.

I repeated: "How did you get the idea about Sam Carr?"

He hesitated before he replied: "I met Sam Carr in the distance. Not everyone gets too close. He's very reclusive. It looks like a dog; he talks through it. He hears it."

"How do you know this?"

Berkowitz screamed: "How? You wouldn't understand!" I can still hear his sarcasm. I tried once more. "How did you get the idea about Sam Carr?"

"I went down there," he mumbled.

"Where?"

"Down the street, where his house was."

"How did you find his house?"

"I saw it," he said, still hesitant.

"You saw it from your window, isn't that so? You live high up on a hill, and Sam Carr lives far down below, possibly two hundred feet in a direct line of vision."

As I spoke, Berkowitz regarded me quizzically, no doubt wondering how I knew all this. I hadn't told him that I had visited his apartment house in Yonkers, and had been shown the small house of the real Sam Carr, down below.

"What did you do then?" I asked.

"I went down and looked at the house and saw his name and address outside the house."

"So you found Sam Carr. He exists in reality."

Berkowitz nodded. He asked me if I had spoken to Sam—

obviously concerned that his whole story was about to unravel.

"Why did you go down to Sam's?" I pursued.

"From my apartment I'd heard some howling and barking, and I wanted to find out what it was all about."

"What happened?"

"When I stood outside Carr's house, I couldn't hear anything, but when I came back to my apartment, I heard a dog barking again."

He told me that the demon voices had become weak and even disappeared when he had been in Florida and Texas. It appeared that the voices came and went depending on where he was, which indicated that he was able to control the demons and their voices, rather than their controlling him.

A psychiatrist often has to investigate a crime beyond the interview with the defendant to determine whether he is fit to stand trial. In this case, I knew I had to look into the matter of the barking dogs. Berkowitz had already convinced the two court-appointed psychiatrists that he had "heard" commands to kill through the barking of dogs. But I had to determine for myself how much those animals were a real presence in his life, and how much a part of his fantasies.

I paid a visit to the Son of Sam's former landlady in New Rochelle, and was surprised to see that she had two dogs tied up in her garden. She told me that when Berkowitz had come to ask about renting her attic apartment, she had told him about the animals and he had blurted out, "I don't like dogs." "Well, take it or leave it," she had responded. "The dogs are going to stay." He took it.

For two months he had lived in that apartment, and the

dogs, who barked frequently, were right under his window. Since then he had been living on the top floor of a seven-story building in Yonkers from which he could often see and hear barking dogs. One was Sam Carr's dog, Harvey. Berkowitz had also shot a neighbor's dog when its barking became intolerable, although he was never found out. Clearly, Berkowitz could have extreme reactions to the animals. On the other hand, to do such a thing also suggests that he did not feel entirely helpless and dominated by the beasts.

I had never seen so many dogs in one place as I did on the streets of that Yonkers neighborhood. The sound of barking never stopped. In fact, I visited every place where Berkowitz had lived as an adult and found dogs in abundance at each location. Whatever Berkowitz had made of the animals in his imagination, it seemed almost that he sought them out. It seemed increasingly likely that he had used the real dogs to create a story to explain his own violent feelings—psychopathic, perhaps, but not paranoid. The demon-dogs did not control him any more than paintings control the artist who painted them.

Finally, for a man who did not like dogs, Berkowitz had a peculiar job in 1976 at a time when, according to him, the demons were already sending him out to kill. He was employed as a night watchman at a large security firm, which assigned him to patrol a warehouse on the West Side of Manhattan. He was accompanied on his nightly rounds by three large dogs.

"I loved those dogs," he told me. "We were buddies. I took care of them, fed them, bathed them." Nevertheless, he admitted, one of them had bitten him, drawing blood.

"What did you do?" I asked.

"I bit him back," he said, laughing.

Berkowitz never mentioned feeling frightened or anxious about his hallucinations; obviously he could tolerate them quite well. And during all my interviews with him, he never mentioned feeling anxious or panicky the first time he had hallucinated. Yet every person I had ever treated who suffered hallucinations had felt terror-stricken the first time it happened.

Genuine hallucinations originate from within the mind; they are not imaginary constructs based on external stimuli. I was satisfied that Berkowitz interacted with the animals on a conscious level, that they were part of his everyday life.

Berkowitz' deep sense of guilt was the final undoing of the demon story. Early on, he told me of his remorse about the killings. With only slight irony, and more relief than he probably realized, he had told the police who took him into custody: "You finally got me. What took you so long?"

Those guilt feelings could be of greater importance in understanding his personality. I sought to illuminate his guilt by probing his unconscious. One day I asked him if he had had any dreams while confined at the hospital. "Dreams?" he countered defensively. "No." Then, "Yes. I dreamed I was swimming in the East River, and that somebody was after me in a boat. I was swimming around Manhattan. I got up on the pier in Manhattan. I was wet and had to change my clothes somewhere, so I went to Gracie Mansion to meet the Mayor, to shake his hand."

He interrupted himself. "It's very noisy here," he complained. "I don't sleep well, but I haven't had bad dreams here. The shower feels good."

Plainly, Berkowitz was in no mood to continue on that

subject. I waited until our next meeting to return to the dream, and particularly to his shaking hands with the Mayor.

"Were you perhaps asking for forgiveness?" I wanted to know.

"I didn't want forgiveness," he declared flatly. "Who needs that?" His voice rose to a scream.

I needed to know if he had any free associations to his dream, and so I pressed on.

"Have you ever seen the Mayor?"

"When I was arrested."

"Where?"

"It was at Police Headquarters. He stopped and looked at me, and then he just walked away."

"How did you feel about that?"

Berkowitz shrugged.

"Did you feel important because he was there?" I persevered.

"No."

"Do you know why he was there?"

"Yes, he was there because of me. He had a press conference."

Berkowitz was trying to divert me from digging too deeply into his dream. Dreams often tell us of our carefully guarded and repressed feelings, and they do not lie. They bring to the surface what is buried in the unconscious. Berkowitz was afraid his dream might expose something revealing, and he was right. I interpreted the dream as an attempt to seek forgiveness from the Mayor, the "head" of the city and thus an authority figure. The person pursuing him in a boat was also an authority figure. Berkowitz' conscience was bothering him; the Mayor's forgiveness might relieve his feelings of guilt for the murders he had committed in New York City. Not surprisingly, from that point on he refused to discuss his dreams.

"Do you think it's possible for a person to talk himself into a mental condition?" I asked Berkowitz one day.

"Yes," he agreed, "you could talk yourself into something; but I didn't do that," he replied, looking me right in the eyes.

A psychosis can't be turned on and off at will. Berkowitz had clearly constructed the demons in order to provide himself with an explanation for his violence. The demons were a product of his conscious, deliberate thoughts, appearing at his beck and call. The hallucinations had not come to him; he had created them.

II

I completed my series of examinations on September 28, 1977. In my report to District Attorney Gold, I observed that Berkowitz' symptoms did not fit any category of mental illness known to psychiatry. His delusions were simply malingering. I also wrote that he had "complained to his lawyer that I hadn't talked much about his delusions or his demons, which had been such an important topic in the other psychiatrists' interviews. Apparently he felt that his distorted beliefs were of such importance that all other topics should be relegated to the sidelines. The purpose of such a tactic should be obvious."

I concluded that while Berkowitz did show some paranoid traits, he was able to stand trial.

Meanwhile, the officers responsible for transporting Berkowitz halfway across Brooklyn to the courtroom where the competency hearing would be held were having second thoughts. The Son of Sam's crimes had hardly endeared him to the people of New York. There had been cries of outrage when, shortly following his arrest, the Criminal Justice Agency, a public-service corporation set up to make recommendations on bail, suggested that Berkowitz should be released on his own recognizance because he had a permanent residence and a steady job. When the arraignment had taken place at Criminal Court in Brooklyn, crowds had massed outside screaming, "Kill! Kill!" Prudence dictated that Berkowitz' exposure to the public be kept to a minimum. So it was decided that the hearing would be held on the prison ward of Kings County Hospital.

On October 20, 1977, the day of the hearing, wind gusted erratically along the wet streets and rolled off the high buildings. These stormy blasts and the pelting rain seemed an entirely appropriate setting for exorcising the Son of Sam's demons.

In the courtroom, artists, seated among the reporters, were busily sketching all the principals. At the back were five rows of chairs for more reporters and a few selected members of the general public. I recognized the mother of Stacy Moskowitz, the last of Berkowitz' victims, sitting among the spectators. If he was found to be mentally competent, Berkowitz would stand trial for Stacy's murder.

As the Son of Sam entered the courtroom, flanked by two guards, everyone strained to see him. He attempted a smile, but his taut, ashen face betrayed him. I wondered if at last he had begun to realize the seriousness of his

141

situation. He was seated between his lawyers. Judge John R. Starkey, a man in his sixties, tall, gray-haired, somber in his black robes, entered the room.

The court-appointed psychiatrists were the first to testify. They played a tape of a forty-five-minute interview they had conducted with Berkowitz. They described the psychotic nature of his delusions and testified that they did not doubt that Berkowitz was insane and incompetent to stand trial.

When it was my turn to testify, I reviewed my initial encounter with Berkowitz, and I told the court that the defendant had read my book *The Murdering Mind*, in which a competency hearing had been discussed. I concluded that Berkowitz' delusions were transitory and situational rather than constant, and that I believed he exaggerated them considerably.

Ira Jultak, in his cross-examination, suggested that his client's murderous impulses were totally out of his control. He cited an incident in which Berkowitz had gone out to the Hamptons, on Long Island, with the intention of committing a murder. In my report I had noted that Berkowitz had returned home without shooting anyone and thus demonstrated that on any given day he did not *have* to kill, even if he felt so inclined.

When Jultak pressed me to admit that the defendant really thought he heard demons speaking through barking dogs, I reminded him that Berkowitz had been virtually surrounded by real dogs, and that when Berkowitz had complained to his landlady about her barking dogs, he had never used the word "demon."

Finally, Judge Starkey spoke:

I am convinced by a preponderance of the evidence...that the defendant is fit to proceed....I think that everybody is agreed that he understands the proceedings against him.

Can he perceive, recall and relate? He can to a great extent. Does he have a rudimentary understanding of the criminal process in the roles of judge and jury, prosecutor and defense attorney? I think that must be answered in the affirmative. Can he establish a working relationship with his attorney? That's been demonstrated. Does he have sufficient intelligence and judgment to listen to advice? Yes, to listen. There might be a doubt as to whether he would take the advice. But that doesn't interfere with his ability to listen to advice....I find...beyond a reasonable doubt, that he is competent to go to trial.

The defense, however, convinced the court that a second competency hearing was in order. The second hearing was set for April 1978.

Again I interviewed Berkowitz and found him showing considerable remorse over what he had done. This recognition of his guilt was important, because such a state of awareness usually reflects a well-integrated ego; he might have been a troubled young man, but I had no more reason now to doubt his sanity than I'd had when I first examined him.

"What happened with the demons?" I asked him.

"They've gone," he answered matter-of-factly.

"Suppose that in the end your lawyers feel you shouldn't plead guilty, that you should claim insanity?" (I was referring to a possible trial, and not the upcoming competency hearing.)

"I won't go along with them."

"Why not?"

"Because I'm the one who gave them the idea of pleading guilty. I told them I wanted to plead guilty in the first place, a couple of months ago."

The result of the second competency hearing was the same as that of the first—that Berkowitz was fit to stand trial. The defense attorneys now counseled Berkowitz to enter a plea of not guilty by reason of insanity. He was also under pressure from his adoptive father, Nathan, for whom a not-guilty plea based on the insanity defense would offer some respite from the horror and tragedy that was unfolding.

But in the end, David Berkowitz' view of himself prevailed. On May 8, 1978, before three State Supreme Court Justices, he pleaded guilty. Sentencing was scheduled for May 22.

On that morning, the door of the courtroom opened and Berkowitz appeared, handcuffed and surrounded by five correction officers. He looked panicky, his eyes wild, and he was fighting his guards, who were trying to restrain him. He was chanting loudly, in a sarcastic singsong, "Stacy is a whore, Stacy is a whore. I'll shoot them all."

The court was in an uproar. Stacy Moskowitz' mother, sitting just in front of me, cried out in anguish, "You're an animal!" and hurried from the room. Robert Violante, Stacy's boyfriend, who had been almost blinded by one of Berkowitz' shots, had to be comforted by his father.

Berkowitz bit one of the officers and twisted the head of another, until at last he was carried back into the anteroom.

As people once again took their seats, someone near me remarked, "Mad as a hatter!" I answered drily, "Not so."

This was theater, with Berkowitz acting and directing. Judge Joseph Corso, who was presiding, responded to the performance by delaying the sentencing until June 12. In the meantime, the judge asked for another psychiatric report to aid in his decision.

I felt that Berkowitz had disrupted his sentencing to maintain his status as the star of the show. No one could doubt that the scene belonged to him.

Prior to his second appearance for sentencing, on June 12, Berkowitz was warned to behave. He was told that disrupting the proceedings would do him no good because he could always be excluded from the courtroom and sentenced in *absentia*, which was the court's privilege. Although he promised compliance, he was given Thorazine, a major tranquilizer, just to make sure. In court, he appeared quiet and docile, but I suspected that that was as much the result of the no-nonsense advice he had been given about controlling his emotions as from the medication. Incredible as it may seem, he yearned for approval; when it suited his interests, he could be a "good boy."

Berkowitz was sentenced to 547 years. He would be eligible for parole in twenty-five years. This was too much for one spectator, a young man sitting behind me, who leaped up and ran to the front of the courtroom in an attempt to grab Berkowitz. The man was seized, wrestled to the floor and carried out, struggling and raging like a trapped animal. During this outburst, Berkowitz was led to a back hallway, where he told a court attendant, "Why didn't you let him get at me so he could tear me to pieces?" I wondered if he would have welcomed the attack as a way to atone for his murders.

Early the next morning, the prisoner was taken secretly to the Ossining Correctional Facility, formerly known as Sing Sing; from there he would be transferred to the Clinton Correctional Facility, near Dannemora, New York, where he was to undergo psychiatric and physical examinations. In July, he spent about six weeks at the Central New York Psychiatric Center, in Marcy, where he was examined again. Finally he was taken to Attica Prison, where he would serve his time, no longer shielded from the reality he had tried to hide from as the Son of Sam.

III

Ordinarily, that would have been the end of my involvement in the case; but it was, in a sense, a beginning. Not long after he was sent to prison, Berkowitz initiated a correspondence with me that has lasted to this day. I subsequently visited him in prison and through these meetings and letters learned more about the psyche of the man who called himself the Son of Sam. Oddly enough, I, the man who had sent him to prison, was to play the role of his confessor.

In retrospect, this strange state of affairs was not totally surprising. Before the second competency hearing, Berkowitz had asked me to tell him if I thought he should plead guilty. I had declined, since that was a matter to be decided between him and his lawyers. But his question had made me realize that he was gaining confidence and trust in me—perhaps because in some sense I was the only person who took him seriously. Now that he was in prison, he wanted me to help him understand why he had acted as he had, and he explicitly authorized me to publish my findings.

In February 1979, Berkowitz announced in a press conference at Attica that he had invented his demon story. A month later he confirmed it once again to me in his first letter, remarking that he had "never thought this demon story would carry out so much." A few letters later, intimating that he had an idea why he had killed, he suggested that I come up for a visit. I went to Attica several times, and Berkowitz made it clear to me that he wanted his story told, and that he did not expect to profit from it.

In all, I acquired extensive notes from the interviews and received more than four hundred pages of typed or handwritten letters from him, a wealth of material to illuminate his personality and his crimes.

Often his letters showed an obsession with guilt. In one fantasy, he had imagined how his day in court should have gone:

JUDGE: Has the jury reached a verdict?

JURY: We have, Your Honor.

JUDGE: Then will the foreman of the jury please read the verdict to the defendant and the court.

JURY: David Berkowitz, we, the people of New York City, find you not guilty by reason of insanity.

DEFENDANT: Wait! I'm the killer. I killed all those people. I shot them with my gun.

JURY FOREMAN: No, David, you didn't kill anyone. Your sick mind was the killer and it wasn't your fault. We all lose our marbles once in a while. Now go in peace and stop tormenting yourself with guilt.

That same letter also portrayed his manipulative nature and his need to be the center of attention.

I knew... that all I had to do was slide "Sam Carr" and the "demons" into the conversation and I'd have him [one of the court-appointed psychiatrists who had found him to be insane] bending over his chair in my direction. Why he'd practically been wiping the tears from my eyes and comforting me, saying, in a sense, "don't fret, don't cry, you're a sick, sick boy."

...And, thank God he listened to it, for it was all I had. Had someone taken it away, then I'd have been standing there stark naked, guilty as ever, with nothing to hide behind, no safe ground, nothing but my own self.

...Others were my little puppets. People to be manipulated. They bent forward when I wanted them to, they talked about the subjects that I wanted to speak of, and they told me just what I wanted to hear—that I was not guilty!...

You, however, wouldn't allow yourself to be manipulated that way. You did stick to your guns. You refused to yield and, as you know, I fought you like an alley cat would fight [another] alley cat—two mates fighting over a lovely feline...

Unfortunately for me, too, I lived a most lonely life in the year before my capture. I was lonely for I had a deep, deep secret that I wanted to share with my friends. It was on the tip of my tongue and I wanted very much to say it: "Hey, I'm Son of Sam."...

I was often tempted to telephone my father, saying: "Dad, have you got a minute because there's something I want to tell you?" Or, I wanted to sit my two precious nieces, one on each [knee], and say: "I know you kids won't believe this but I want to tell you that I'm..."

Guilt-ridden, exhibitionistic, self-aggrandizing, manipulative—he was all of these. But I still did not have an answer to the most important question: why had he killed?

I concluded that the force which had driven Berkowitz to homicide was what it so often is in cases of murder: the sexual drive. People like to think of sex as a means of expressing love, but we know that it is intimately associated with hateful, even murderous inclinations. Love and hate are closely intertwined, and the distance between them is short. The sexual force—through jealousy, competition, envy and a wish for revenge—may not only initiate but also stimulate, mobilize and ultimately maintain murderous impulses.

Having always suspected that Berkowitz did not have a "normal," satisfactory sex life, I was hardly astonished now to discover that in fact, his sexual development had been distorted. While sexual development is not the only determinant of human behavior, it is certainly one of the strongest.

As a Freudian psychoanalyst, I believe that a great deal of our adult behavior is influenced by early sexual development, and by how successfully we have passed through the psychosexual, or Oedipal, stage of childhood. Freud theorized that unless we move beyond our childish competition with the same-sex parent for the affection of the opposite-sex parent, we will remain dependent and emotionally immature. While psychologists of other orientations will not necessarily work within this framework, certainly all of us agree that poor family relationships in early childhood are bound to have lasting effects unless problems are resolved at some point through therapy or very diligent self-help.

In reply to my question about his sexual fantasies, Berkowitz wrote: "I envision myself as a lover who is passionate, well endowed, and is able to please my mate in giving her a multitude of orgasms. I picture myself as one who has no qualms about performing oral sex with the female genitals. In fact, I would enjoy it very much. I would also be able to prolong (delay) my ejaculation for hours until my partner has numerous orgasms and is begging for mercy." Berkowitz was often preoccupied with oral sex to the exclusion of genital intercourse ("...most often my fantasy involved oral sex between heterosexual couples"). To me that suggested an immature sexual development. He preferred petting and fondling to adult genital intercourse, exhibiting the sexual propensities of a child of five or six—an age at which children fondle and examine their own and each other's genitals and display themselves. Berkowitz' obsessive calling of attention to himself was a reflection of this voyeurism and exhibitionism outside the sexual realm.

In his adult life Berkowitz had masturbated as a substitute for sexual intercourse. "I always fantasize about girls," he told me. "Now I cannot go to sleep unless I masturbate first." His neurotic shyness had kept him from the company of real women. In his daydreams he always had a girlfriend, but there was little reason for him to leave the security of fantasy for the uncertain world of real women, where rejection was always a fearful prospect.

In the sense that Berkowitz had built a wall between himself and the feelings and experiences that most adults have—however painful and difficult they may sometimes be—he had cut himself off from an important realm of human reality. We all begin to fantasize between the ages of three and five, and we continue that activity throughout our lives. Creative fantasies—daydreaming—stimulate the imagination and can prepare us for some later action. But Berkowitz' daydreaming served only as a repository for wishes he felt helpless to fulfill. Rather than being a stimulus to action, they became, for the most part, a substitute for living.

Berkowitz' sexual shyness was rooted in the circumstances of his childhood. He was told when he was three that he was adopted, and although he could not possibly have understood its full significance, he was old enough to realize that in some sense he did not completely belong to his family. His adoption became a central concern in his life, and the notion of being different also engendered in him a feeling of ambivalence toward the rest of the world. He developed a deep and abiding feeling of estrangement; there was, he felt, something basically wrong with him.

His adoptive mother, Pearl, became the focal point for his ambivalence, although Berkowitz was reluctant to discuss it. When I brought it up at the first competency hearing, he interrupted the proceedings with a passionate description of how he had cried at Pearl's grave. He had never been sure of the authenticity of her affection, and he particularly noted his mixed feelings about the times when she had kissed him: did it mean she really did love him? At an early age, he generalized his uncertainty about his adoptive mother to include all women. Feeling that the affection of the first woman in his life had been untrustworthy, he would not try for another woman's love.

Berkowitz' feelings of alienation and the effect of the loss of his birth mother were aggravated when Pearl died of cancer when he was only fourteen. If he had equated love and affection with rejection and ambivalence before this unhappy event, they now became joined in an intimate bond, and a poor preparation for adult relationships.

Against this backdrop of an uncertain love, Berkowitz reenacted an age-old drama; but here, as elsewhere in his life, he could not work through the conflict successfully. In the classical Oedipal confrontation of childhood, Berkowitz stumbled. "I resented my father because he had my mother," he bluntly put it to me. He recalls being asked to leave his parents' bedroom, where the only television set happened to be. "What are you going to do, kiss?" he recalled saying to his father in those situations. He laughed as he related this to me. His father's reply was usually "David, your mommy and I have something to talk about."

Berkowitz needed to identify with his father; he had to think of himself as effective in his relationships with women. But he felt as ambivalent about his father as he did about his mother; the identification could not take hold, and he found himself unable to grow up.

Incapable of feeling real love and affection toward women, uncertain of his own masculinity, Berkowitz had nowhere to go with his sexual feelings. The result was frustration and a festering malevolence toward all women. "I began to hate girls," he told me in an interview. He began to be "troubled" by his fantasies, which were all either sexual or violent. He felt that he was perverted. Yet even here, ambivalence (and repression) showed through. He wrote: "When I fantasize myself having sex with a woman, it's never violent. But in my mind, sometimes I have the desire to cause bodily harm but not while having sex. My violent fantasies are miles apart from my heterosexual fantasies." Or so he thought.

He did not understand that violence often plays a role

in sexual fantasies. In the disturbed mind, however, these feelings, sex and violence, literally fuse. Divergent or dissimilar emotions become associated with, connected to or merged with each other. Such was the case with Berkowitz, in whom sexual feeling was overtaken by violence.

Berkowitz told me that he had "fantasized about shooting a woman for a long time," and although he had no one particularly in mind, he knew it would be a pretty woman. The way that his stymied sex life was caught up in his murderous activities became clear when he described his last crime, the attack on Stacy Moskowitz and Robert Violante.

He was both voyeur and participant in their lovemaking, taking his pleasure vicariously. When he reached the point where he wanted to take part in the act, he fired his gun. He was transfixed as he pulled the trigger, sexually engaged as he took a life. Enormous gratification came with the discharge of the gun; with the release of the tension, he felt an orgasmic exhilaration and a great sense of well-being.

Emotionally a child in a man's body, sexually thwarted, bewildered and vengeful for having been left by both his mothers, Berkowitz was a person who lived with a volatile and deadly mixture of conflicting thoughts and feelings. He finally dealt with his confused sexuality by shooting women, penetrating them in a symbolic and impersonal way, thus obviating the need for intercourse. "I regard the female as dangerous," he told me. Had any woman who crossed his path known his thoughts, she would have done well to view him in the same way.

Berkowitz really grew up with two sets of parents: Pearl

and Nathan, and the shadowy, fantasy figures who had given him up at birth. Pearl appears to have had little understanding of, or empathy with, David—possibly because he was not her own flesh and blood, but more likely because she just couldn't handle him. Early on he was obviously a troubled child. He writes: "It frightens me to look back and see what I was and what I became.... Why didn't someone see the signs?" He was constantly in trouble in school, set numerous small fires and generally exhibited many of the traits of a disturbed youngster. Nathan was usually out attending to his business, a father figure who reportedly involved himself little with his son. I wondered whether there had been one single person or incident that finally tipped the scale, that turned this pathetic and thwarted human being into a mass murderer.

David Berkowitz had a burning desire to recover his past. In 1975, with the assistance of ALMA (Adoptees Liberty Movement Association), and after six months of hard work, he managed to find his birth mother and half-sister in Queens, New York. His natural father had been dead for some time, but that did not stop Berkowitz from fantasizing that he must have been "wild-tempered, greedy, impatient." Meeting his mother and sister was, he had told me when we first talked at Kings County Hospital, "a very warm, nice experience." He also expressed great pride in having discovered their whereabouts.

Given the ambivalence that characterized every aspect of Berkowitz' life, however, I expected he would have the most conflicting feelings of all concerning this discovery. Not only had he been given up: his half-sister had been kept. Now he had further evidence of rejection, and he saw Betty, his natural mother, as the root cause of all his unhappiness. The loving, long-lost son was, inside, seething with vengeance and hatred, and the lid was about to blow.

Not long after this reunion, he attempted his first murder. His primary hunting ground was Queens, not coincidentally the place where he had found his mother and sister. It was as though in his activities as the Son of Sam, he sought to repay all the women in his life for his pain and confusion. (Was he, perhaps, unconsciously trying to ensure, through his killings, that other women would not get pregnant and bring forth more David Berkowitzes into the world?)

Once he started to kill, it became easier. His eight shootings took place over the course of a year. They occurred at intervals of one to three months in a pattern that suggests a repetition compulsion. As with a drug addiction, the first time was a little fearful, but he became more accustomed to it as time went on, and eventually it became almost routine.

Berkowitz thought of himself as a kind of Jekyll and Hyde. "It is interesting to note my changes in behavior and actions during the daylight hours and at sunset. They were two opposites. At night I hunted. In the day, I helped. I became vicious and lethal at night to people I never knew before and who I just met by chance. On the other hand, during the day, I was kind, friendly, courteous..."

I realized that never before had the inner conflicts in the personality of a mass murderer been so documented. All the more reason, I felt, that labels such as "multiple personality" should not be too quickly applied. In contrast with the case of a true double, or multiple, personality, Berkowitz exhibited no amnesia or loss of memory in any respect. On the contrary, he had clear recall of the details of all his crimes. What he had was a character disorder. Like Garrett Trapnell, he was a psychopath, not a psychotic.

But Berkowitz did live in two different worlds, and the fact that he was conscious of it in no way lessens the terrible consequences of that split for his victims, nor mitigates his responsibility for what he did to them. The ambivalence that shadowed the life of David Berkowitz had terrible consequences when it emerged into the world in the avenging form of the Son of Sam.

In the end, David Berkowitz saved some of his greatest hatred for himself. A Jew, he converted to Christianity and groveled in his sinfulness. It may also have been his own way of abandoning his mothers, both of whom were Jewish. He seemed to revel in the wrath of an angry God, although at the same time he was genuinely fearful of this deity, who for him was actually a projection of the father/authority figure he had never come to terms with. Berkowitz called himself "Die Schmutz"—the dirty one.

In the end, nobody will punish the Son of Sam more than David Berkowitz. I was not surprised to read the headline on July 11, 1979: "SON OF SAM KILLER SLASHED IN THE NECK AT ATTICA." Berkowitz had refused to name his attacker; he even tried to make light of the whole incident, referring to his assailant as a "pain in the neck." But I thought there was something more to it, and I brought it up the next time I saw him:

"Were you afraid of being attacked?" I asked him.

"No, not afraid. I sort of willed it."

"Were you conscious that you willed it?"

"I'm not sure." His uncertainty indicated to me that there had been an element of wishing.

"When you say that you willed the attack and you expected it, did you feel that you deserved it?"

"Maybe. I don't know."

But later he wrote to me:

It was quite an experience—a positive one in the long run. Plus, this scar gives character to my face....I now feel secure and that there is a sense of justice in the world. There is really a law of cause and effect. I've always wanted punishment, the punishment I deserve—I love being punished. So, this was it. I've been trying to expiate my sins for so long. This just felt so good (mentally). It felt almost as if I was miraculously cleansed for the time being.

7
THE TORMENTED
TEENAGER

Jack Casin, sixteen, and his girlfriend were driving in his family's car when it crashed head on into another car. A young mother and her infant died in the accident and three other passengers were severely maimed. Local newspapers described Jack as a murderer, and he received anonymous hate mail. Jack was sentenced to five years' probation and his learner's permit was revoked.

The subject of this story, a fairly typical teenager, was not a "criminal" in the sense in which Gary Trapnell, David Berkowitz and many others were, although he was convicted of a crime. Rather, he was the protagonist in a kind of tragedy in which misunderstanding and thoughtless actions changed several lives forever.

Mr. and Mrs. Casin [all the names in this chapter are pseudonyms] came to see me to ask if I would treat their eighteen-year-old son, whom they described as sleepless, fearful and depressed. Since the accident Jack had been under treatment twice by psychiatrists, but if anything, he had sunk deeper into his depression. It seemed odd that with therapy and the passage of time he not only had made no progress, but had even retrogressed. I agreed to see him.

Two days later, Jack, a good-looking young man, slowly entered my office. He haltingly told me that he felt totally apathetic about his life.

"Why so unhappy?" I asked.

He didn't really know, although he mentioned, almost casually, that he had been involved in a head-on collision two years earlier. When he said that, he looked away.

After a pause, he filled in the terrible details: "Two people were killed, three injured."

"Were you hurt?"

"I didn't realize it then, but my face and neck were bleeding. The police took me to a hospital and called my parents. They came. They didn't know I had a girl in the car. I was dizzy and upset...."

Only sixteen at the time of the accident, Jack had been driving with a learner's permit. His fourteen-year-old girl-friend Sharon had been with him, although her injuries were minor. In the months that followed, he felt confused, and he had what he described as very angry feelings toward everybody, toward the whole world. When I tried to get him to expand on that cryptic revelation, all he would say was that "There was something wrong."

When I saw him the next time, I noticed that he tilted his head to the right, trying to hide the scar. Almost as soon as the session started, he said, "I've been covering up something. It's with me every morning....I try to accept it."

"Can you be more specific?"

"My father is fighting me." He apparently hadn't heard me. "I'm pretty confused."

The confusion was present as he spoke to me. He rambled quite a bit, skipping from topic to topic without much feeling. It is not unusual for a patient or defendant to wander this way. Such random statements can, however, be quite useful to a psychiatrist. In fact, he is specifically trained to make the most of this kind of "raw" material.

"I am friendly, altruistic, try to help people," Jack went on. "I take on things that are more complicated than I think they're going to be. I'm helpful; I want to feel I can handle it, but other people don't think I can. I failed my road test twice. 'You're a bad kid.' I heard it from inside, from my mind."

He stopped and was quiet. Although he gave the impression there was more that he wanted to say, he seemed unable to go further.

The subjects he had touched upon were obviously related: strife with his father; confusion; his belief that he himself was essentially a good person; the negative judgment of others; a failure in a test; a judgmental voice that he had internalized. They all pointed to a deep sense of guilt, although it was obviously not simply that, because there was also the unexplained anger.

After several sessions it was apparent that he was putting a great deal of energy into concealing something— from himself, I thought, as much as from me. On the other hand, I sensed that he also wanted to open up and talk freely, which boded well for the ultimate success of a course of therapy.

As the facts about the accident were filled in over the next several weeks, I got a better idea of what he was up against. He had been arraigned a mere three weeks after the accident, while he was still dazed and unable to cope with the enormity of it. Two weeks later, a grand jury had indicted him on several counts, among them third-degree assault and criminally negligent homicide. Sharon was the only eyewitness who testified. The stories in the newspaper and the anonymous letters had left him dreadfully confused and depressed.

Jack had pleaded guilty to all counts of the indictment. Because of his age, he was accorded youthful-offender treatment, and two months later was sentenced to five years' probation, with his learner's permit revoked. Considering the grisly toll from the collision, one might have expected him to be relieved that he had not been imprisoned; but that was not the case. Something was eating at him.

Since Jack seemed to find it difficult to talk about himself while he faced me, I suggested he make use of the couch, facilitating, I hoped, the easy expression of his thoughts, feelings and free associations. I would modify classic psychoanalysis—in which the analyst seeks to let the patient wander wherever his psyche will take him—intervening when necessary to offset the paralyzing effects of his depression. Jack was willing to give it a try.

We started slowly. He had flickering reminiscences of the collision. Then he seemed to be getting at something about Sharon. Then he skipped to academic problems in school. When he got back to Sharon, I was at least able to learn that her parents were divorced and that she had been in therapy herself.

Jack revealed that at the age of fourteen and a half, he had driven his father's car when he was out of town. "I could have had an accident," he remarked. "I was scared;

I knew how serious it was; I wasn't a careless, reckless kid, but I was challenged to try and get away with it."

Then he began to offer some possibly significant information. He spoke of Sharon's odd behavior after the fatal collision: "Sharon was freaking out.... She came to my house after the accident, was willing to give herself to me. 'Let's do something together,' she said." He couldn't figure it out. He knew that at that point she was already going out with somebody else. He paused, and in the silence I thought about Sharon, wondered what she was up to.

"Just before the accident I turned on the radio," he went on. "Her kneecap was hurt. Right side of the car had splintered glass..." Then he stopped, just as he seemed to be on to something.

Jack recalled being at the filling station where he worked on the morning of the accident. Sharon had come over and the two of them had driven off to get some pizza for lunch. "I had one accident the Saturday before," he told me. Nobody had been injured, but he had been emotionally shaken by that earlier accident. "I had too many things on my mind....I trusted her," he rambled. "When the accident happened, I was hurt and I said to her, 'Go get help.' She took off, went back to the service station. I didn't realize how serious an accident it was. I had blocked out that she was in the car.... She talked about it at school. I was surprised. I had told her to leave for my own protection."

That last remark—"told her to leave for my own protection"—was probably a slip of the tongue. But at this point its meaning was ambiguous. Why would hiding the girl's presence in the car protect him?

Then he mentioned a priest he had been talking to once

a month, who had asked him, "Do you know what you did?" "He brainwashed me, made me feel guilty," Jack observed. Although he spoke softly, I sensed a good deal of anger simmering beneath the surface. Jack seemed to have had enough of authority figures who made him feel guilty.

Any kind of therapy usually involves going over the same subject several times. Over a period of time, the accretions from each session build on the original story until the details become clear and the entire picture is brought into focus for the patient as well as the therapist.

At our next session, Jack returned once again to the accident:

> I think I remember I turned on the radio....I was trying to get comfortable, worried and scared about going out with the girl. I had a lot of confidence in her. I trusted her enough to let her handle situations.
>
> When I drive I concentrate on keeping control of the car. I wasn't that experienced. I wouldn't really have time to turn on the radio. The last thing I remember clearly is passing another car. I can't recall how fast the other car was going or the position of its passenger....I don't remember it vividly, but I do remember that our car went over the yellow line, out of control, into an oncoming car. I heard the noise—hitting the guardrail; I don't remember seeing it. The car swerved a bit; the back end of the car hit the guardrail. After the accident the car was never examined for mechanical defects.

Now that he was able to deal with the incident at some length, I encouraged him to stay with it. I got him to concentrate on where and when the collision had occurred. As he related that information, he shifted rest-lessly on the couch.

"A lady yelled dirty names at me, called me a mur-derer," he added. "I wasn't myself. There was something with my brain. Concussion...I was unconscious..." he said, apparently trying to grasp some essential but cur-rently unreachable fact about the crash. "...whether it was a police car or an ambulance," he continued, just short of coherence, the chaos of his thoughts mirroring the scene of the collision.

But then he did say something clearly, and it seemed to irk him. Sharon, who had left to get help, had returned with Mike, another employee from the gas station, al-though they had both remained in Mike's car, and "she never came forward to admit she was involved in it." By then, the accident scene was honeycombed with police.

A fourteen-year-old could not be expected to cope eas-ily with the blood, the dead and the dying. It would have been easy for her to panic in the midst of the moaning and screaming, the sirens and the police. Still, something about her behavior bothered me. Her attitude immediately following the accident contrasted sharply with her be-havior a few days later when she visited Jack at his home. Was that loving concern, or perhaps an expression of some guilt that she felt? He had not yet been entirely forthcom-ing about her, I sensed.

As time went on, Sharon's role in Jack's psyche and the accident itself loomed larger. One day he related a dream: "I was in the car with a girlfriend. We were both intoxi-cated. The car started pulling out of the parking lot. The police came. I knew I wasn't going to be treated fairly. But the police arrested me, and the next thing I knew I was sentenced to the electric chair, and I was electrocuted. The last thing I knew was that I couldn't understand why I was so evil. In the dream I said something to the effect 'You weren't supposed to be there in the first place, to be driving, so it serves you right.'"

He was still stuck in his passivity and the self-punishing, masochistic fantasies reflected in the phrase "it serves you right."

Given the fact that he was dwelling on his guilt feelings, it did not surprise me that he now jumped to the subject of his father's attitude toward what had happened. Punching out the words in a staccato fashion, he recalled his father's anger and how he "was disgusted when he learned I had a girl in the car."

But almost in the same breath, Jack said, "There was a hole in the...windshield; a wound on my neck—red. Sharon banged her knee," almost as if his unconscious were trying to put together the pieces of a jigsaw puzzle.

Then the subject shifted back to his father once again. He recalled his father's "wild" reaction when he had come upon Jack and Sharon having sexual relations. He described Mr. Casin as a strict parent who "was always checking up" on his son. "He never let up." It wasn't in the boy to assert himself. In a resigned voice, he said, "He has a right to control me, to tell me what to do." If he had listened to his father, Jack thought, he would never have gotten himself into this fix.

Just before the end of the session, Jack returned to his dream. In commenting on its vividness, he unwittingly demonstrated the marvelous inventiveness of the unconscious mind. "I was electrocuted," he reiterated. "I was shocked when I woke up." He didn't realize that he had made a very dramatic and telling pun. He might indeed need to be shocked before he really awoke.

As Jack delved further in the circumstances of the accident, his feelings surrounding it and his relationships with his father and girlfriend, it seemed easier for him to recall his thoughts and feelings at the time of the accident.

"The police thought I was alone in the car. When she split after the accident, I didn't even remember that she had been in the car. I can't explain how my mind was," he told me, trying to make sense of what had happened. "I knew I was in trouble, so I rationalized, for some reason, that Sharon wasn't in the car. And when I did remember, I didn't want anyone to find out. I figured I wouldn't get into as much trouble that way; it wouldn't look so bad."

Jack's sense of guilt over his relationship with Sharon, and his concern over what others might think, must have been a heavy burden if it could color his thoughts even when he was in shock right after the accident. In our next session, he cast more light on the interconnection between his feelings about her and about his father.

Mr. Casin did not like Sharon, and a few months before the accident he had demanded that Jack have nothing more to do with her. At about that time Sharon's father had called Jack's home at midnight, to see if she was there. Angry and upset, Jack's father had run up the stairs to check his son's bedroom, only to find him there alone.

Sharon was a troubled girl. One time, Jack related, she had tried to run away from home. She had come to his house, but "we made her leave." A year after the accident, her family had moved out of the neighborhood. Was it only a coincidence that after the accident they had moved from a place where they had lived for so long?

At this time I had a long interview with Jack's father. A devout man, Mr. Casin taught a weekly religion class to high school students. Sharon had been one of his pupils before the collision. Oddly enough, after she moved away she returned to the neighborhood once a week to attend the class. She gave no indication that she had been suddenly seized by a religious fervor, and her motives seemed open to question. It was clear to her that Mr. Casin did not like her, and he had tried to prevent his son from seeing her; what was she up to?

In the light of her presence in the car at the time of the accident and her odd behavior since, it was obvious to me that she felt very guilty about something. She might have imagined that she had been a party to some transgression. But one thing was certain. By putting herself in a position where she was constantly being confronted by Jack's father, a man who had only negative feelings about her, she was, compulsively and repetitiously, subjecting herself to a good deal of self-punishment.

While Jack had loved and trusted Sharon, he also feared and resented her because she was an added source of friction between himself and his father. His loyalties were in conflict, and the stress and trauma of the accident had accentuated that division, making it all the harder to deal with the painful memories of that fateful day.

Mr. Casin's feelings about Jack were also ambivalent. The father recalled rushing to the hospital when informed of the accident, finding his son with a bloody bandage on the front of his neck. Jack had at first refused to have the jagged wound stitched, and his father had had to give his permission for the medical team to sedate his son so that the sutures might be put in.

Jack's father expressed obvious concern about him as

168

we spoke, but he was also hypercritical; almost punitive. He felt protective toward the boy, but had also been terribly swift in his judgment of Jack's behavior at the time of the accident. He clearly did not trust Jack.

At this point in his treatment, Jack's free associations were spilling out in a distinctive pattern. First some thoughts, fantasies or memories of the collision, then often something about his judgmental father, then back to the accident. In one session he remarked; "I don't think we were going fast. Maybe fifty, sixty miles an hour; maybe forty-five." He said that quickly, then turned around to look at me to check my reaction. Seeing me sitting there silent and impassively listening, he again became absorbed in his thoughts.

"I was angry, but didn't say anything," he remarked.

"At whom?" I asked.

"At my father. He was always after me. I couldn't express myself. I was afraid of him. He wanted it his own way. He was always looking over my shoulder."

I realized that Jack's increasingly severe depression was due at least in part to the fact that the accident had increased his already excessive passivity. He was now even more dependent on his father than before. Since his learner's permit had been revoked, he could get around only if his father or mother drove him. The day of the accident, he had taken the family car without permission — a rebellious act which, ironically, resulted in the curtailment of whatever independence he had been able to develop.

As his feelings about his father came pouring forth among his recollections of the accident, his mind seemed gradually to focus more sharply on what had happened that day.

One day, at the end of a long pause, I asked him, "What's on your mind?"

"I think of the accident every day. A friend who has known me for a long time told me after it happened that he...feels I suppressed the truth of the accident, that I let other people get the best of me." Immersed in his thoughts, he said, almost to himself, "Why did she split after the accident?"

After another pause: "[I knew] he would be very angry when he learned I had a girl in the car, disgustingly angry....There was a lot of pressure on me and I had to handle it somehow." Then he stopped. When he continued, he said insightfully, "Maybe I set myself up to get into trouble and try to get out of it, but this time there was no way out. She shouldn't have been with me, and I should have been at work."

By now he was agitated; he cryptically referred to all the bad dreams he had been having. I didn't press him on that. It had been a long, searching session, and he needed a rest, a chance to mull things over.

In clarifying a defendant's state of mind, a psychiatrist must play the role of detective. But when treating a patient over a long period of time, the patient himself must be a detective along with the doctor. Indeed, the ultimate success of the course of treatment depends on whether or not the patient is finally able to put all the pieces together. As far as I was concerned, a possible outline of the final picture had emerged, but it was necessary for Jack to make the connections that would lead us both to clarity.

In our next session, Jack recalled what it had been like going back to school after the accident: "Sharon had built a wall around herself. She had told everyone what happened, and she wouldn't let me say anything." He described his ambivalent feelings about the affection she offered him at this time. When he expressed his anger at her initial refusal to get involved, she had said that she had to protect herself—an explanation that did not satisfy him. Meanwhile, he had to face the rest of the world. "It was a complete drain, day in and day out. Everybody knew what had happened—*they* told *me*. I got the feeling they knew more about it than I did." He felt that everybody was judging him and that only by "taking the whole blame" could he get other people off his back. His mother showed compassion, but his father had a different attitude. "He gave me shit."

In the next few months it became evident that Jack's resistance to dealing with the reality of the accident had lessened to a point at which I could push him to try to recall—consciously and out loud—exactly what had happened at the time of the crash.

"You told me that you remember your car went over the yellow line, that it went out of control. And that the back end swung around and hit the guardrail. Why did you go over the yellow line?" I asked him.

"It happened on a long left curve." He stopped to gather his thoughts. "The car...the back of the car, I think, hit the guardrail and went over to the left."

I asked him to draw a diagram of the crash scene. It showed that his car had crossed the middle line and collided with the oncoming car.

In response to another request, he drew a diagram of the windshield of his car after the collision.

"And you went through the windshield on the right side—not the left?"

"Yes, that's it."

Sharon had said that the car was speeding—Jack had

171

DAVID ABRAHAMSEN, M.D.

told me that previously. Now I reminded him of her statement, and it jarred him. He suddenly recalled that the
speedometer on the car had been broken, so how did she
know they were speeding? He looked determined, less
depressed. Was he finally awakening to something? He
toyed again with the notion that the story he understood
was inaccurate. However, he was not yet ready to confront
whatever was still hidden, and he drew back from what
to him must have seemed like a precipice.

In the next few months of therapy, he consolidated the
gains he had already made. He also began to express more
anger at the rapid way in which the authorities had disposed of his case. I reinforced his feelings, telling him
that I too was surprised at the speed with which he had
been arraigned, been indicted, pleaded guilty and been
sentenced, without anyone's really investigating the circumstances of the crash in any detail.

One day he said to me, "I couldn't tell them the girl
was in the car, and that I wasn't driving, because I didn't
know. But the police could have figured it out."

"How?"

He began to stammer.

"Go ahead," I encouraged him. But instead of answering
my question, he told me about a dream:

"In the courthouse I said to the police, 'I wasn't driving.
Taking into consideration the circumstances and the suffering, I feel confident at this time I was not driving.'

"'How can you change your story?' the policeman asked
me.

"'I was emotionally high-strung.'

"The police said, 'It will ruin our reputation.'

"I continued, 'I don't care about your credibility. No-

172

body has ever given *me* a chance to be the way I was. I was not driving. It is a shame you did not come to the right conclusion on your own!'"

We dream about what we wish for or about what we fear. While Jack's free associations and dreams had been pointing increasingly to a belief that he had not been driving when the accident occurred—and thus had been suffering needlessly—I could not yet say with *absolute* certainty that that was the case unless he could be sure; there was always the outside chance it was a wish. In addition to the trauma of apparently having caused death and injury, Jack had been branded a murderer, placed on probation and lost the privilege of driving. Now he was involved in a $3 million lawsuit filed on behalf of the survivors of the collision. He would have good reason to wish that he had not been driving that day—if he had, in fact, been behind the wheel.

Mr. Casin was now constantly reminding me that his son would have to appear soon to testify at a hearing in the suit, but I put him off, explaining that not only was Jack not yet in any condition to testify, but certain of my findings had already cast some doubt on his culpability. For that reason, the hearing was delayed.

I needed a bit of physical evidence before making up my own mind on the matter—and the police supplied it: photographs of the smashed-up car. The hole in the windshield was on the right, just where I had suspected it might be, not even close to the driver's side. Jack was surprised when I showed him the photos. His mother told me that she had picked slivers of glass out of his hair for two weeks after the accident. Generally, the driver of a car will not go through the windshield: the steering wheel will prevent it. The story was falling into place.

I asked Jack how he had let himself be pushed into confessing to something he had not done. He said the scene of the accident was horrifying. "The people were violent, screaming at me," he recalled. "I never had a chance to tell my side; I had to listen to what everyone else said to me." In court, it was the same. He was put under enormous pressure and did not know what he was doing: "I didn't understand the implications and consequences when I pleaded guilty. I didn't say very much because I didn't understand what had happened. There wasn't anyone I could sit down and talk with. I would get probation, I was told. But I didn't know my learner's permit would be taken from me, and that I couldn't drive for five years."

He went on to describe the moment when he had told the judge that he was guilty. "I *was* guilty in many ways," Jack said. "I shouldn't have taken the car, I shouldn't have let the girl drive, I should have obeyed my parents." It almost sounded as if, to appease his sense of guilt for all sorts of matters totally unrelated to the case, he might at that time have confessed to anything.

Jack was now prepared to appear at the hearing in connection with the lawsuit, and he stated flatly for the first time that he had not been driving the car at the time of the crash. He could not remember precisely when he had changed seats with Sharon, but there was no doubt in his mind that she had been behind the wheel.

There was also no doubt in my mind that the young man who had come to me with a mysterious depression almost two years before had been feeling that way because he had been misled into confessing guilt for an accident he had not caused.

Given the way the police and the court had handled the case, I believed a terrible miscarriage of justice had occurred. On the basis of the new evidence, the case had to be reopened.

Solving Jack's legal problems was not easy, but we were now in a position to begin. I obtained copies of the reports by the psychologist and psychiatrist who, at the direction of the court, had examined Jack three months after the accident so that I could see how they had assessed his mental state at the time of the crash. Their conclusions were a reflection of the sloppy way the case had been handled by the authorities involved.

Jack...appears quite upset by the accident, denies responsibility for the automobile collision.... [He] feels that his father has set expectations too high for him to achieve and, in general, is a demanding parent. Jack feels that his mother, although emotionally upset over the accident, has been more supportive than his father during the ordeal....He is a good student, poor in impulse control.

It was the examiner's impression that Jack had some difficulty relating because of this nervous anxiety...in addition to his anxiety and impulsivity, Jack's defense mechanisms at the present time are characterized by a great deal of denial and intellectualization....

Projection techniques indicate...Jack is a mildly depressed, anxious young man who has a great deal of potential for impulsive acting-out behavior.... The difficulty he has had in the past in successfully relating to his parents is hypothesized to be at the core of his confusion. Jack seems quite angry toward his parents for his inability to...obtain...support and structure from these authority figures....He is a moderately severely disturbed youngster who demonstrates a significant need for therapeutic intervention as well as additional support and structure from adult authority figures around him...[an] insightful youngster who seems cognizant of his own disabilities and would probably be quite willing to accept help with his own emotional confusions.

He was confused, all right—but at least part of that had come from the "support and structure" he had received from the "adult authority figures around him." The person writing this report had simply taken Jack's confession of guilt as the truth and attributed his denial of blame to simple psychological evasion.

When I checked the emergency-room records of Jack's admission to the hospital on the afternoon of the accident, I saw something else that should have been reflected in the psychiatrist's report. Jack's blood pressure had been very high—the diastolic pressure, at 100, and a systolic pressure of 140 had, in fact, been pathological for someone his age. This symptom indicated that the boy was under terrible strain and stress and was certainly in no condition to respond to questions from the police. Nor did the mental-health professionals who examined him mention in their reports that Jack's initial confession had come at a time when he had just suffered a concussion.

The blow to the head had caused Jack to have retrograde amnesia—a memory loss that extends backward to include thoughts and feelings which predate the trauma that precipitated the amnesia. That accounted for the greatest part of his confusion and subsequent depression. "Something was wrong," he had told me when he first came to see me. Something was wrong indeed.

In preparation for reopening the case in court, I got in

touch with the lawyer who had originally defended Jack and informed him of what I had discovered. He responded immediately with a letter stating that he was now in a position to reassess his earlier evaluation of the case and that the guilty plea had been wrongfully entered.

I filed a report with the county district attorney detailing my findings. I concluded that the concussion had seriously interfered with Jack's capacity to reason for a period of time following the accident. On the day he had pleaded guilty, his state of mind had been such that, by reason of "mental disease or defect," he was incapable of knowing whether or not he had been driving the car—thus satisfying the requirements of the state law on the changing of a judgment. Jack could not possibly have understood the implications and consequences of his guilty plea, and therefore the court should reconsider and vacate the earlier judgment.

I took it upon myself to secure a good lawyer for Jack; and I hired a specialist in accident investigation to testify on the circumstances of the collision. He conferred with the district attorney's office about Sharon's testimony to the grand jury and came up with some interesting information:

> ...There are several discrepancies in Sharon's version of the accident. She told the Grand Jury that she was a passenger in the auto with Jack, and that when she saw him hit the guardrail, she slid down underneath the dashboard in anticipation of a crash. Later on in her testimony, she stated that she slid down in the seat and braced her knees against the dashboard and her back against the seat. She related that she ended up on the floor and Jack went

through the front windshield on the passenger side. In either case, she should have sustained injuries requiring medical attention....

There is no mention of Sharon accompanying Mike [the boy with whom she returned to the crash site] back to the accident scene.... The police report does not include Sharon's name as a witness nor as a passenger in the auto.... The only report the District Attorney had was that on the afternoon of the next day, the police received an anonymous phone call that there had been a girl in the auto with Jack Casin, [giving] them Sharon's name and address. When the police tried to question her, Sharon's father contacted their attorney and refused to allow Sharon to be interviewed. That same evening, Sharon appeared at the hospital emergency room complaining of injuries she had received in the auto accident of the previous day.

Sharon was now offered immunity from a charge of perjury for her previous testimony if she would be more forthcoming now, but she was willing only to pass along a brief statement through her lawyer: "Jack Casin went through the passenger window. I was lying across the front seat. I lost consciousness, and when I came to Jack was sitting in the driver's seat."

I suggested that Jack and Sharon be offered the opportunity to take a lie-detector test. She refused, but he was glad to take it, and it confirmed his story.

While we waited for a final hearing, Jack continued in therapy. He recalled that he had just been giving Sharon a chance to learn how to drive. For the first time he described himself as "innocent," at least in the legal sense, although he was aware that he must bear some responsibility for the tragedy. "I cannot wipe out the remorse or guilt I felt for the family in their tragedy," he said quietly. "...It is haunting me."

At the hearing I presented my findings on Jack's mental and physical condition. There was no cross-examination. Within two weeks the judge dismissed the original indictment, and the worst of Jack's nightmare was over.

Freud once wrote of secrets that "In the case of the criminal, it is a secret which he knows and hides from you, but in the case of the hysteric, it is a secret hidden from him, a secret he himself does not know." The secret that Jack had hidden from himself had been devastating. In bringing that secret to consciousness, he had freed himself from an unjust legal burden and gained hope where before there had been only despair.

8
PROFILE OF
AN ASSASSIN

For many Americans, the world changed on a grim November day in 1963. The assassination of President John F. Kennedy appeared to mark a turning point from the optimistic, progress-filled years that followed World War II to a time of internal strife and violence. Suddenly guns and death were everywhere, assassins stalked world leaders, murderers lay in wait for the rest of us.

We may risk making too much of symbolic turning points in history. Kennedy had not been the first American leader to be killed, and street crime did not begin in 1963. Certainly the good old days of the late 1940s and the 1950s gave us, as well the Korean War, the witch-hunt for domestic subversives and a good deal of racial violence.

Assassination itself was certainly nothing new. Our history books are replete with political killings: the assassinations of Julius Caesar, Jean Paul Marat, Abraham

Lincoln, the presidents of France and the United States and the king of Italy at the turn of our own century, Archduke Franz Ferdinand and Mahatma Gandhi, to name just a few.

But whether we are dealing with the deed in ancient Rome, medieval Persia or our own time and country, one thing has always been consistent: the presence of some link between victim and assassin—an idea or ideal that one stood for and the other detested, despised and loathed.

The killing of President Kennedy, however, did not fit this pattern. Despite some odd political connections, Lee Harvey Oswald made no political claims when he was arrested. He will never know what we might have learned about him because he himself was gunned down only two days after the President's assassination by a man who seemed to have no more link to his victim than Oswald did to Kennedy.

The misfits who have shot their way into the history books since Oswald all seem to have wished primarily to call attention to themselves, seeking notoriety for its own sake. Assassination, we discovered with the fatal shootings of John Kennedy, Robert Kennedy, Martin Luther King and John Lennon and the attempts on the lives of Governor Wallace, President Reagan and President Ford, could be an end in itself as much as a means toward an end.

I believe two factors are substantially responsible for this increasingly familiar and horrifying phenomenon. The first is our easy access to firearms. A gun is one of the most impersonal of weapons. The person who shoots someone achieves all the emotional release of murder without having to be physically close to his (or her) victim. Rage can be vented without hands being bloodied—the killer can keep his distance and maintain intact his alienation and isolation.

The second contributing factor is the increasing influence of the mass media. Television in particular has become so pervasive that all of us, to some extent, receive our notions of reality from it. For the person whose sense of separation between fantasy and reality is weak, the publicity given an assassination attempt—successful or not—can trigger the acting out of hostility along paths already made familiar. Now it is possible for anyone to make the six-o'clock news.

Statistics bear this out. From 1960 to 1963, the number of threats against the lives of prominent government figures in this country averaged about 200 a year. But from 1964 to 1968—the years immediately following the assassination of the President, years in which violence of all kinds was daily fare on the television news—the annual average jumped to 1,100—an increase of about 550 percent.

But numbers alone do not tell the whole story. Increasingly, these threats were marginally political or not political at all. What type of person were we now dealing with? How much could we generalize about the personality and behavior of the individuals threatening to kill public figures?

In 1968, the increase in criminal, racial and political violence was such that the National Commission on the Causes and Prevention of Violence was enjoined to study the problem, and I was asked to testify on the increasing number of threats being made on the lives of prominent figures. I had examined a dozen men held on such charges, and in my testimony I profiled one of the more illustrative cases.

"Joe" (a pseudonym) had called the FBI in Washington and announced that he was coming down to "kill one of the big wheels." In a second call, he repeated his threat and even described the clothes he was going to wear when he arrived; he also said that he had a gun. On the appointed day, federal agents boarded trains running between Boston and Washington and apprehended him, recognizing him from the accurate description he had given of his appearance.

When arrested, he claimed that two Latin Americans had offered him $200 to kill the President. He also said, falsely, that he had been in the Marine Corps. Later he claimed that he had been drinking just before he made the trip; but he was not intoxicated at the time he was taken into custody.

An only child, Joe was the offspring of a domineering mother and a father who had been arrested twice for drunken assault. His parents' restaurant took up almost all their time, leaving their son alone for much of his childhood. Not surprisingly, he became a troubled youth, and a still more troubled young man. His mother blamed Joe's problems on the Army, which he had entered after dropping out of high school. He had begun to drink to excess at that time, and from this point on, his life was a series of failures: going AWOL three times from the Army, quitting his job, leaving his wife and children to return to his mother's house, suicidal feelings and two admissions to psychiatric hospitals, the second time under an assumed name. He told the doctors that he had terrible headaches resulting from a head injury he had suffered in the Army.

He also claimed to have been brought up in an orphanage.

Following his arrest for threatening to kill the President, Joe was put in yet another mental hospital for observation, where he was described as tense and frightened, an alcoholic and a liar. When I examined him, I discovered that he had one overwhelming need: to attract attention to himself.

So fragile was his sense of self-esteem that he even sent himself telegrams stating that he had won a big prize in a contest, so that he could flash them in front of his acquaintances. Another time, when Joe discovered that the police were looking for a missing person, he reported having him. In fact, the missing man was already dead.

Although Joe was passive and dependent, he had vivid fantasies of omnipotence. The tension between Joe's passivity and his fantasies of omnipotence became potentially dangerous when he felt threatened. Self-destructive, given to histrionics and grandiosity, Joe found an attempt to kill a public figure—sabotaged in advance by his calls to the FBI—the perfect way to vent his rage.

Although Joe and the other men I studied differed in the details of their cases, they all shared some general characteristics. One could expect to find, in some measure: grandiose ambitions, recurrent revenge fantasies, impotence, desire to be in the limelight, isolation, self-hatred and self-destructiveness, helplessness, dependency, fearfulness and excessive sensitivity to criticism. The typical family situation was a weak, unassuming or absent father and a domineering mother.

The men I examined ranged in age from twenty to forty, except for one who was over sixty. The language they used in their threatening letters and calls was generally straightforward: "I am going to assassinate the President," "I am going to kill the President." When caught and confronted with the evidence, these men consistently denied, rationalized or minimized their threats. One said there had been a "misunderstanding"; another claimed to have been drunk; still another simply refused to interpret his letter declaring that he would kill the Vice-President as particularly threatening. One man couldn't understand what all the fuss was about. "They had power," he stated with sweet reason; "why couldn't I?"

Their responses are like those of a child who, when caught stealing, denies the truth even to himself. The child and the would-be assassin believe the lie. They have feelings of omnipotence, a kind of control over reality: I want something to be true, and therefore it is true. The person with a fantasy of great power denies feelings of being completely helpless. The fantasy is gratifying, while the reality is too painful.

Revenge was a common theme in these men's threats and fantasies. Often they had been rejected as children and projected their rage at their parents onto public officials. Quite frequently, too, they had been subjected to sexual stimulation by their mothers—something these defendants shared with sex offenders. Typically, their mothers had been seductive, but also withdrawn. The pattern seemed to be one that alternated between tenderness that went beyond manageable bounds and wounding aloofness. Real attention and love had seemed always out of reach, and the child had been left confused, enraged and vengeful.

What distinguished this group from other criminals was their interest in world events. These men read newspapers and books. They saw the world as a chaotic place which, in their visions of omnipotence, they must "clean up." Much of the outer turbulence they saw was, of course, the projection of their own state of mind. And in their grandiose and omnipotent fantasies of changing the world through assassination, they were begging for help for the dependent child within them. Ostensibly, they were out to kill government officials; in truth, they wanted to be cared for, nourished and protected by those authority figures, who replaced the parents who had abandoned them.

II

Lee Harvey Oswald shared many of the characteristics of these men. But *he* carried out his plan; he succeeded. But I was puzzled. Had Oswald done what he had intended to do?

In the first decade following President Kennedy's assassination, hundreds of books and articles examined the killing. Concern over the many loose ends approached something of a national mania, and the conspiracy theory was widely discussed. Two decades later, we are in a better position to make some sense of the tragedy.

Each of the three Presidents killed before Kennedy— Lincoln, Garfield and McKinley—was murdered by a man who confessed to his crime and explained his reasoning. But in the two days that Lee Harvey Oswald was in police custody, he made no confession or statement as to his motivation. In the twelve hours of uninterrupted questioning by Dallas police (who for some reason did not record the interrogation), he steadfastly denied having shot at the President. Nor could his wife, Marina, his mother, Marguerite, or his brother, Robert, all of whom

talked with him during this time, move Lee Harvey Oswald to admit to the shooting.

I was greatly intrigued by the strange circumstances
surrounding President Kennedy's death. Although neither I nor any other psychiatrist was ever able to examine
Oswald after the murder, psychiatric testimony on the
nature of the crime and the kind of mentality such a criminal would exhibit was solicited by the Warren Commission, and I was one of those called in for consultation.

Something about the story of the crime as reconstructed
through eyewitness testimony and police reports has continued to bother me. The questions raised about the incident so often seem to have been the wrong questions.
Not that all the initial areas of inquiry weren't important
and worth pursuing: whether Oswald had acted alone or
had been part of a conspiracy was crucial to the investigation. But all the evidence suggests that Oswald was a
loner, withdrawn and secretive, not the kind of person
who becomes part of a conspiracy.

More interesting, though, were Oswald's motivation and
intention. What did he think he was doing, and why? In
that respect, Marina Oswald's testimony to the Warren
Commission seems especially important. She was asked
about her husband's attitude toward the President:

Q. Did your husband make any comments about President Kennedy on that evening, of the twenty-first?

A. No.

Q. Had your husband at any time that you can recall
said anything against President Kennedy?

A. I don't remember any— [his] ever having said that.
I don't know. He never told me.

She also went on to say that when she heard that her
husband had shot at the President, it "was surprising. And

188

I didn't believe it. I didn't believe for a long time that Lee had done that...."

Q. Why did you not believe this?

A. Because I had never heard anything bad about Kennedy.

In itself, this exchange proves nothing. Given her husband's secretive character, one would not have expected him to discuss his plans for killing President Kennedy. But it was interesting that Marina had not picked up the slightest sign of animosity on Lee's part toward the President, and that for her, Lee's shooting of Kennedy was a tremendous shock. I studied closely the twenty-six volumes of the Warren Commission report, particularly Oswald's "diary," his letters to his mother, wife and brother, and the psychiatric examination done on him when he was thirteen years old. I also communicated with those who had personal knowledge of his family background, especially people who might shed some light on the role of Oswald's mother and wife in shaping his state of mind at the time he fired the shots.

In a case in which the evidence was fragmentary and the killer had been killed in turn so soon after his crime, I believe that a thorough examination of Oswald's background might suggest his state of mind at the time of the assassination and provide a reasonable hypothesis for just what might have motivated him.

Lee was born on October 18, 1939. His father had died two months before his birth. His mother, Marguerite Oswald, constrained by poverty, first sent Lee and her two older sons to their aunt, and then had to break up the family. Lee's brothers were put in a Lutheran boarding home, while he returned to his mother.

Marguerite rented rooms in her house to a couple with

the understanding that they would care for Lee while she worked. She came home unexpectedly early one night to discover that they had been beating her child. She decided that Lee must join his brothers in the boarding home. It was the day after Christmas.

Lee never adjusted to life at the home. The age difference between himself and his brothers precluded closeness with them, and his mother's habit of taking him out to live with her for short periods of time effectively prevented him from developing relationships with the other boys.

Lee began to believe that nobody cared about him, probably assuming he was a burden, a "bad" boy. He was also never able to come to terms with his father's death, and may have imagined that somehow the man had not "wanted" to be with him. Marguerite's feelings about Lee appear to have been confused: at some times she left him with others; at other times she overloaded him with attention and affection.

A youth probation officer who saw Oswald at the age of thirteen, when he and his mother were living in New York, has said: "The mother worked. I got the feeling that she was so wrapped up in her own problems she never really saw her son's. She spoke of her comedown in life after the death of Lee's father. She didn't mention that she had remarried. I got the impression that what Lee needed most was someone who cared, especially someone who could represent a father to him. He was a small, lonely, withdrawn kid who looked to me like he was heading for trouble."

Young Oswald withdrew into himself. He became suspicious, distrusting all authority figures. He developed a rigidity of character to protect himself against what seemed a very unfriendly world. Obsessed with himself, Oswald shared the narcissistic, attention-seeking traits his mother had in abundance. As in the case of other would-be assassins, Oswald's self-image swung from omnipotence to debilitating helplessness.

The dossier on Lee's behavior confirms his troubled state. At the age of nine he threw a knife at one of his brothers, and a few years later threatened to stab his brother's wife. In his early adolescence he struck his mother on several occasions. He was frequently truant from school. Oswald was court-martialed twice in the Marine Corps, and once shot himself in the hand "accidentally." While in the Soviet Union he attempted suicide. In 1963 he shot at the right-wing activist General Edwin A. Walker. Nor was Lee Harvey Oswald a good family man; he was a wife-beater.

On the surface, Oswald appears to have been political, but his politics seems to have lacked any personal commitment. His public pronouncements manifest a spirit of exhibitionism—words for the importance of their sound rather than for communication. His professed commitments to Cuba and the Soviet Union are expressions of psychological projection and identification rather than ideological engagement. Fidel Castro was an authority figure upon whom Oswald could project his confused feelings about authority figures. He once told his wife that he himself would one day be prime minister of Cuba. His "defection" to the Soviet Union was more an abandonment of the country that, like his parents, had failed to sustain him than a commitment to Communism. By a leap of the imagination, Oswald perhaps conceived that Mother Russia would do for him what his own motherland (and mother) had not.

A central theme in Lee Harvey Oswald's life was his difficult relationships with women; and central to that had been his pathological interaction with his mother. In some striking ways, Marguerite was the perfect model for her very imperfect son. She was extremely narcissistic, inflexible, possessive, contemptuous of authority, exploitative and cruel. In fact, in awarding her third husband a divorce in 1948, the court commented that she had been "guilty of excesses, cruel treatment and outrages."

To Marina, it was clear that Lee "did not love his mother." She "told him that he should be more attentive" to her, "but he did not change." In all fairness to Marguerite, she had had a wretched life, filled with emotional and economic deprivation, and had learned early to control her family with guilt and manipulation. The relationship between mother and son was one of love/hate; the hate largely generated by the twisted way in which love was expressed. For much of the first ten years of his life—at least for those periods when he was not living elsewhere—Lee Harvey Oswald shared his mother's bed.

During that time Marguerite was married, and for a young boy, such an arrangement provides sexual overstimulation in the extreme. The consequence for him was revulsion toward sexual intimacy. He developed an acute shyness toward girls, and during his marriage to Marina he was constantly troubled by impotence.

Rejecting and seductive in a maddeningly alternating cycle, Marguerite made him both dependent on and terribly fearful of her. Although he tried to escape his mother's influence, he never found a creative and successful way of accomplishing that.

The Marine Corps served as a refuge for a time. But

Marguerite even managed to reach him there: she had him discharged on the ground of hardship when she injured her nose, claiming that he had to come home and support her. Lee lasted at home for three days. He gave her $100 out of the $1,000 he had saved while in the Corps and then departed, against her bitter complaints.

When Oswald left for Russia, he wrote to his mother: *"It is difficult to tell you how I feel. Just remember this is what I must do. I did not tell you my plans because you could harly [sic] be expected to understand....I will write again as soon as I land."* The word "love" never appears in the letter, and in fact she did not hear from him again until two years later when he thought she might be able to help him leave Russia.

Oswald returned to the United States with a Russian wife, Marina, who thought at least some of her new husband's behavior rather odd. He would often withdraw, becoming "quite a stranger. At such times it was impossible to ask him anything. He simply kept to himself. He was irritated by trifles." He could also become violently jealous, at which times he often beat her.

When Marina visited Lee following his arrest for the murder of President Kennedy, he told her "that everything would turn out well. But I could see by his eyes that he was guilty," she recalled. Guilty, but of what? I wondered.

Just as in the criminal cases I had dealt with directly, it seemed to me that the best answer to the question of motivation and intent would be found in combining the physical evidence and the psychological history of the defendant as best as we could.

Given that we must depend to some degree on speculation, it is important to note two incontrovertible facts about Lee Harvey Oswald as a sniper. The first is that he was an excellent marksman using good equipment. Garland G. Slack, a customer at a rifle range frequented by Oswald, observed his accuracy on at least two occasions: the two weekends prior to the assassination. Slack recalls being impressed by the "tight group," or close cluster of bullet holes, that Oswald made on his target.

According to Malcolm Price, the operator of the rifle range, Oswald was test-firing a gun with a telescopic sight on the weekend of November 9–10. Price looked through the sight and was impressed by its clarity. On the other hand, we know that the FBI, for a month, repeatedly test-fired the gun Oswald used in the murder of President Kennedy and could not duplicate what appeared to have been the assassin's accuracy. They found that the telescopic sight and the rifle could not be aligned on the target adequately because the scope was mounted off center. The equipment itself was fine, but it simply wasn't assembled precisely enough. This, then, is the dilemma. Oswald was an excellent marksman, but the scope on the murder weapon was poorly aligned. I have concluded that Oswald's shots were *not* accurate and that he never hit his target.

One of Marina's first reactions to news of the shooting was to ask if Mrs. Kennedy had been hurt. Knowing at first hand of her husband's vengeful feelings toward women, did she, without knowing, arrive at the truth about his motives?

Oswald had never known a father, and all his rage was focused on his mother—everything he hated neatly wrapped up in one package. Oswald's voracious reading of political literature had oriented him toward the public realm, so killing Jacqueline Kennedy, *the First Lady*, would have been a source of immense gratification for him. Not only would he have dispensed with "Mother": he would also have been the first man to kill a President's wife, thus assuaging his desperate need to feel important and special.

When Oswald vehemently denied shooting at the President, he was in all probability telling the truth. Given his mental state at the time, he was not refusing to admit to a crime; he just could not bring himself to acknowledge a mistake. He had been a failure all his miserable life. Now he was being charged with one of the most infamous deeds of the twentieth century, and he would go to his grave knowing that he couldn't even get that straight.

9
OF MIND
AND MADNESS

On March 30, 1981, outside the Washington Hilton Hotel in Washington, D.C., John W. Hinckley, Jr., attempted to assassinate President Reagan. In the ensuing scuffle, three men, one of them the President, were seriously wounded. At his trial, Hinckley was found not guilty by reason of insanity. Could there be any justice if Hinckley could get away with this craven act?

With the decision in the Hinckley case, the whole concept of criminal insanity was called into question. Opposing psychiatrists at the trial had worked hard to discredit each other's application of the criminal-insanity law. To the public, the law and its application seemed arbitrary and eminently unjust. Some even called for its complete abolition.

I agreed that the verdict had been a mistake, but I was not comfortable with the public outcry against the *insanity* plea. The main problem is not necessarily that our

197

laws aren't tough enough, although some could be improved; much of the fault lies in careless interpretation of existing laws. It is an ancient concept that there must be a clear and decisive relationship between criminal intent and a criminal act, and for good reason: if a person could not appreciate the significance of what he was doing, and was thus not responsible, how can punishment have any value? We are then left with the problem of determining responsibility—defining what we mean by insane, and applying that definition to specific cases. This is a complicated and subtle matter.

We all have antisocial fantasies—Goethe wrote that there was no crime for which he could not find the tendency in himself—but only a few persons act out those fantasies. And of those, still fewer really cannot help themselves. Under what specific circumstances, then, does it make sense to say that antisocial acts have followed *inexorably* from antisocial thoughts?

The demarcation between the willfully malicious criminal and the offender who is simply not responsible is hazy; when we are dealing with human beings the lines cannot easily be drawn. But criminal insanity must be definable for the purposes of law enforcement.

We must have some boundaries, then, as to what is normal, what is abnormal. More important, we need to articulate what is in the gray area, the continuum between the two ends of the spectrum. We must establish criteria to determine which criminal should go to prison, which belongs in a hospital. The public is losing patience with offenders who avoid prison by saying that the devil made them do it. But while the criminal-insanity law has clearly been abused, it is also in our interest to maintain its use

198

in some form. I believe it is important that the public know what the law is, how it is applied and how it might be improved.

II

When a defendant claims insanity—whether only at the time a crime was committed or also while he is in custody—a determination must be made about his state of mind. We must first determine whether that person can be brought to trial: does he understand the charges against him, and can he cooperate with his lawyer in preparing a defense against those charges? It is possible for the accused to be adjudged competent to stand trial and yet later, at the trial, be found not guilty by reason of insanity at the time the crime was committed.

The present standard for judging competency, known as the Dusky Rule, does not require any judgment as to a defendant's mental condition at the time a crime was committed; it simply asks: Does the defendant understand his predicament at the present time? Does he have the intellectual capacity to reason; can he use language and communicate effectively; are his thoughts organized; does he have self-control; can he establish a working relationship with an attorney and appreciate legal advice; and, finally, is he stable enough to undergo the rigors of a trial without having a physical or mental breakdown? For example, Robert Jett Van Horn may have suppressed his memory when he killed his wife. But as long as he was mentally and physically competent, his trial could proceed. On the other hand, a former boxer accused of fraud was, at my suggestion, declared incompetent to stand trial because he was confused, disoriented and paranoid—he suffered from an organic brain disorder, no doubt the result of taking too many punches in the head. It was impossible for him to satisfy the standards set by the Dusky Rule.

Sometimes, the competency hearing turns out to be the whole drama. Such was the case with David Berkowitz. The Son of Sam lost his power when the attorneys were unable to convince a judge that their client was so helplessly controlled by his demons that he couldn't possibly be brought to trial.

A plea of not guilty by reason of insanity, entered at the time of trial, is another matter entirely. Now we are considering the defendant's state of mind at the precise time of the crime, and the issue here is one of responsibility, will and control. The M'Naghten Rule, which I referred to in the Van Horn case, although somewhat modified over time, is still the standard. This rule as amended by the State of New York holds that a person is not responsible for criminal conduct if as a result of mental disease or defect he lacks substantial capacity to appreciate the wrongfulness of his behavior or to act within the requirements of the law.

At first glance, this may look pretty simple. The rule asks if a defendant can tell right from wrong. But the application of the rule is not that simple. In New York State, for example, a commission of which I was a member worked for several years to improve and refine the definition of insanity, and one of the most important changes we made was to add one word: "*appreciate.*" Did the defendant have the ability to appreciate the wrongfulness of his deed? We felt this would grant the court some leeway by enabling it to make a distinction between mere verbalizing and a deeper comprehension of the act. In the early 1960s, the American Law Institute adopted a similar position on the criminal-insanity plea.

As with any legal precedent that has been in effect over a period of time, not every attempt to modify it has taken hold. The Durham Rule, for example, a modification first enunciated by Judge David Bazelon in a case in the District of Columbia, has fallen by the wayside. This rule held that the accused was "not criminally responsible if his unlawful act was the product of mental disease or mental defect." This may sound virtually the same as the M'Naghten Rule, but there is actually a world of difference. The problem it creates involves the nature of the causal connection between the mental condition and the act. How diseased does one have to be for the criminal act to have been determined by the mental condition? Under this rule, a defense attorney had merely to show that his client was mentally aberrant; if the defendant's behavior was sufficiently bizarre, acquittal could be gained. It was not necessary to prove that the person specifically could not know the nature, quality and wrongfulness of his act.

Unfortunately, in actual practice, the M'Naghten Rule is often applied as if it were the long-since-discarded Durham Rule. I remain deeply concerned about the frequent confusion among so-called "experts" over just what conditions do deprive a person of free will and thus compel him to commit an unlawful act. The law is specific: the person must have known the wrongfulness of his misdeeds and been able to obey the law. The law says nothing about strange conduct, outrageously bizarre behavior or

201

even extreme viciousness. The rule asks only if a person had the ability to be responsible for his acts, not whether his behavior would make you nervous if you found him sitting next to you on a bus.

In essence, we must distinguish between a person manifesting a character disorder (a psychopath) and one who manifests a thought disorder (a psychotic). A person may be antisocial, exhibitionistic, narcissistic, alienated, isolated or violent or display any combination of pathological traits to the point where he might be legitimately regarded as psychopathic, but still have the capacity to control his behavior. He may act out those feelings; the question remains: did he have the option of *not* acting on them? Everything else is courtroom melodrama.

A psychotic person is, in modern parlance, "out of it." His thinking is in the realm of magic, and his fantasies totally distort reality. His delusions are "true"—that is, he sincerely believes them and acts as if they were reasonable interpretations of what is going on in the world. Such a person will probably be unable to appreciate the significance of a wrongful act and should not be placed in a prison.

There is, unfortunately, no clear demarcation between states of mind. Labels such as psychopathic and psychotic have their uses, but the forensic psychiatrist has to be careful that in his efforts to get a handle on a case, categories such as these do not become a kind of magical thinking themselves. The specifics of the defendant's state of mind, history and behavior are at question, not which heading can be most conveniently applied to him.

John Hinckley's behavior was bizarre. He had, for example, a pathological need for attention. This would be sufficient to absolve him of guilt in his criminal act only if it can be shown that his behavior was beyond his control, impulsive, reckless. But Hinckley had not only stalked Reagan; he had also carefully followed President Carter. His behavior seemed, in fact, quite calculated.

The jury in the Hinckley case was given two choices: Hinckley had been either sane or insane; no provision was made for his having been borderline but still able to appreciate the wrongfulness of his crime. Under the circumstances, one might have hoped for a hung jury. For a time two jurors held out for conviction, but they eventually changed their minds, and John Hinckley was sent to a hospital instead of a prison.

No matter what criteria are used, there will often be a subjective element in assessing criminal responsibility. When does a person's fantasy begin to take control of his behavior? When is such a person, finally, not himself?

I have worked with two very different cases involving criminal insanity which help to clarify the issue. One concerned an average man with what seemed to be an odd quirk; the other involved a person with a grievance that turned him into a "Mad Bomber."

III

The owner of an plumbing-supply store in the New York metropolitan area called me one day at the behest of his lawyer. The merchant, whom I will call Harold, was in trouble because he had failed to file income-tax returns for several years. He said that he could not pay his taxes because it was impossible for him to determine precisely the size of his inventory. It seemed a strange excuse for tax evasion. Businesses estimate inventory all the time.

When I asked him if he could be at my office early the next morning, he said that that would be no problem—he was up every day at 2:30 A.M., at the latest. "You see," he added, "I have to check on my employees, and some of them come in about four A.M., and I have to be in the store, going over papers…" Diligence with a vengeance, I thought.

There was nothing in the nature of his business that required such hours; Harold just liked them. He obviously didn't get to see his wife too often, but the short, stocky merchant told me when he came to see me that he was happily married, with six children. "Isn't that enough?" he added.

Harold told me that he was depressed because the IRS wouldn't believe that he couldn't take a satisfactory inventory, even when he asserted that there were hundreds of thousands of items to be counted. To my suggestion that he could make an estimate, he replied that that wouldn't be honest.

I learned from other sources that Harold was a noted philanthropist and was much liked and respected in his town. "I have tried to do good," he said. "I don't have much money. You see here what I have. This is the only pair of shoes I have; the only pair of pants; the only jacket." He pointed to each as he noted them. But he lived in a large house and operated a good-sized business, I reminded him. Surely he could afford to dress better. He wasn't impressed with my reasoning.

Harold said that a year previously his fuse box had

malfunctioned, shorting out the whole house. He had felt he had to repair it himself because there was no one else around who could do it. Never having tackled such a project before, he went to the library and studied the matter. Do-it-yourself is a fine notion, but since he was such a busy man, this seemed to reflect some kind of mania. His complaints about the toilet in his bathroom that had not worked properly for a long time appeared to be no more logical. He was oblivious to my efforts to make some connection between that and his plumbing-supply store, which, I was sure, could yield the necessary replacement part quickly enough.

It didn't take much of this kind of conversation to determine that Harold, although a respected figure in his community, and an obviously generous and likable fellow, was monumentally obsessive and compulsive, unrealistic and a truly dedicated masochist who lacked insight into his behavior. Legal proceedings had already been instituted against him for tax evasion, and another psychiatrist and I would soon be testifying in his behalf. Harold fitted perfectly the requirements for being adjudged criminally insane. Not only did he sincerely believe that he had done nothing wrong: he thought he had demonstrated exceptional honesty. And he could no more bring himself to estimate an inventory count than he could walk off a cliff. There was the M'Naghten Rule, clear as day.

But there was a problem: how could I get a jury to accept this? Harold came across as a harmless oddball; the jurors would be looking for a lunatic. Here was the Hinckley situation in reverse: Harold didn't seem to be crazy enough. The other psychiatrist agreed with my analysis, but would describe Harold as schizophrenic, a true psychotic. At the trial he made an excellent presentation, although I wasn't sure the jurors understood his testimony.

I had discussed the case with my wife, telling her how senseless Harold's behavior seemed, and she had suggested that "senseless" should be the key to my characterization of his actions. That's the way I handled it. The strongest psychiatric terms I used in court were "compulsive" and "unrealistic." I depended on a long recital of the details of Harold's peculiar way of life to convince the jury that this man was simply not all there.

The case seemed clear enough to me, but the jury was less certain. It was not until after three hours of deliberation, a deadlock, then more discussion that they returned with a verdict of not guilty by reason of insanity. Harold was required, of course, to pay his back taxes, which he did, and psychiatric treatment was recommended. I felt that justice had been done.

If we had to place Harold somewhere on the broad spectrum from sane to insane, I would classify him as psychotic—although that might not seem terribly convincing or accurate if you compared him with some of the dangerously deranged offenders. Tax evasion is certainly a far cry from murder. Nevertheless, the law is very specific in its guidelines for a finding of criminal insanity, and Harold's thoughts and behavior fitted neatly within those lines. That he didn't rant and rave, lose his memory, tear his hair out or bang his head against the wall was irrelevant. Under the definition of the law, he was insane.

The next case involved a man whose actions and image differed considerably from Harold's, although he was in fact as mild-mannered as the plumbing-supply dealer. Like the Son of Sam, he was a menacing presence in the New York area. Unlike David Berkowitz, however, this man never actually killed anybody, although he managed to stay at large for a decade and a half while he went about his "business." On November 16, 1940, a bomb was discovered at the Consolidated Edison Company, the utility that supplies New York City with gas and electricity. It did not explode, nor did another bomb found near the company's headquarters almost a year later. A few months after the second bomb, the police received a strange note, printed in block letters. It said: "I WILL MAKE NO MORE BOMB UNITS FOR THE DURATION OF THE WAR. MY PATRIOTIC FEELINGS HAVE MADE ME DECIDE THIS. LATER I WILL BRING CON EDISON TO JUSTICE. THEY WILL PAY FOR THEIR DASTARDLY DEEDS...." The note was signed "F.P."

In the next four years, similar missives were received by department stores, hotels and *The New York Times*. Since no bombs were associated with them, and there *was* a war going on, they received minimal attention. From 1946 to 1950 there were no letters. But in March 1950 an unexploded bomb was discovered in Grand Central Station. Bomb-squad detectives identified it as the same type that had been left at Con Edison years earlier. A few months later another explosive was placed at Grand Central, and this time it went off. In the following months several more unexploded bombs turned up around the city, one of them under a seat in a movie theater. Just before Christmas, *The New York Herald Tribune* received a block-lettered note stating: "HAVE YOU NOTICED THE BOMB IN YOUR CITY? IF YOU ARE WORRIED I AM SORRY, AND ALSO IF SOMEONE IS INJURED, BUT IT CAN'T BE HELPED. CON EDISON, THEY WILL REGRET THEIR DASTARDLY DEEDS.... [I] WILL PLACE MORE UNITS UNDER THEA-

207

TER SEATS...." Again, it was signed "F.P."

Although the police tried to minimize publicity surrounding the rash of bombs in order to prevent panic, there was little they could do, since the explosives were being placed at random in public places. Soon a bomb exploded at Radio City Music Hall, injuring four people, two of them seriously. By the mid-1950s the newspapers were making regular reference to the "Mad Bomber."

By 1956, public pressure was mounting for the apprehension of the Mad Bomber. That year he visited the Brooklyn Paramount movie theater, leaving behind a bomb that injured three people. He also sent a confused letter to the *Herald Tribune* in which he accused the press of persecuting him: "WHILE VICTIMS GET BLASTED, THE YELLOW PRESS MAKES NO MENTION OF THESE [?] GHOULISH ACTS. THESE SAME GHOULS CALL ME A PSYCHOPATH. ANY FURTHER REFERENCE TO ME AS SUCH OR THE LIKE—WILL BE DEALT WITH." He concluded by stating that his life was "DEDICATED TO THESE TASKS. I MERELY SEEK JUSTICE." The signature was the familiar "F.P."

The police, suspecting that a disgruntled former employee of Con Edison might be the source of this terror, pressed the utility to search through its old personnel files for possible leads. Months later, the Con Edison files finally yielded the right folder. George Metesky had worked for the United Electric Power Companies, later taken over by Con Edison, from 1929 to 1931. Ironically, his supervisors had described him as a person who cooperated and followed the rules. In his last year of employment he was injured by an explosion while on the job. Complaining of headaches and fatigue, he had retired to Connecticut, where he lived with two unmarried sisters who supported him.

Metesky's arrest, unlike his career, was undramatic. When picked up, he asked the police, "Do you think I am the Mad Bomber?" He was as mild-mannered and cheerful when he was brought in. When questioned about the meaning of "F.P.," he answered, "Fair Play."

The Mad Bomber seemed mad indeed to all those who spoke to him. The general feeling was that he was psychotic, suffering from paranoid delusions. Two psychiatrists at Kings County Hospital, where Metesky was taken initially, declared him unfit to go to trial. Judge Samuel Leibowitz, who was to preside at Metesky's hearing, wanted another opinion, and he asked me to examine him.

Metesky was at Bellevue when I met him. He was wearing a bathrobe, and with his wire-rimmed glasses, neatly combed short hair and friendly smile, he fitted The New York Times description of him as a "beaming church deacon." Metesky was polite and seemed to be trying to answer my questions to the best of his ability. However one cared to categorize him, he did understand the charges against him and was able to cooperate with his defense. According to the standards set by the Dusky Rule, I found him capable of standing trial, and the judge agreed.

On the other hand: during the Mad Bomber's trial, I testified that he was criminally insane and could not be held responsible for what he had done. There was nothing contradictory in that; as I've noted, the requirements for a judgment of competency for trial have nothing to do with the evaluation of the defendant's state of mind when he committed his crimes. Metesky *was* capable of standing trial and he *was* insane.

At that point, I ran into some trouble from Judge Leibowitz, who felt that anyone who could go around planting bombs for so long must have had more than a little method in his madness. In response to the judge's misgivings, I pointed out that Metesky had carried out his "tasks" under delusions that Con Edison was persecuting and insulting him. He had been out to avenge acts that were solely the product of his imagination, and he truly had not grasped the consequences of what he was doing.

Metesky was found to be criminally insane and was sent to Mattaewan and then to Creedmoor state hospitals—from which he was released seventeen years later, an old man who no longer presented a threat to others or himself.

A quirky electrical-supply dealer turns out to be legally insane; a "Mad Bomber," clearly a certifiable lunatic, is adjudged fit to be tried for his crimes—although the verdict at his trial is that he too was not legally responsible for his behavior. Neither case followed a direction the average person might have predicted. There is so much more to this problem of criminal responsibility than just whether or not the defendant appears to be "crazy." The law is specific in setting out the reasons for excusing a defendant from going to trial, or committing him to a mental hospital instead of sending him to prison if he is found not guilty by reason of insanity. I believe that our present laws on criminal insanity are quite adequate and fair when they are interpreted carefully and responsibly.

IV

The abuse of the criminal-insanity law by clever attorneys and psychiatric experts has engendered a growing sentiment for stricter treatment of mentally impaired offenders. Proponents of the "guilty but insane" verdict suggest that such offenders be sent to prison instead of a psychiatric hospital, but with the proviso that since mental condition had *something* to do with the commission of the crime, sentencing should be determined accordingly. But this begs the question of responsibility. If the criminal knew what he was doing and could have acted differently, then his mental quirks cannot be considered mitigating factors. And if he literally could not help himself, what is the point of imprisonment? Clearly, the concept "guilty but insane" is contradictory—insanity and guilt are mutually exclusive. They are two distinct facets of mental functioning. In insanity there is no connection with reality. Only someone with a connection to reality can have a sense of guilt and be held morally responsible.

From time to time objections to the insanity defense have been so strong that attempts have been made to strike it down altogether. Most recently, and notably, former President Nixon in 1973 decided to solve the problem of the insanity defense by proposing to abolish it entirely. Fortunately, his efforts came to naught. At the time of this writing new attempts are being made to abolish the insanity defense.

While establishing someone's guilt or innocence by reason of insanity cannot be determined by a formula, there are, as mentioned earlier in this chapter, established criteria for ascertaining legal insanity.

Unfortunately, under our adversary system of justice, a lay jury must often contend with psychiatric experts arguing against each other. It is extremely difficult for someone without expertise in psychology to choose between them. When a lay person is asked to make a judgment regarding physical illness in a negligence or malpractice case, he is presented with concrete scientific evidence from which to draw a conclusion. In a case involving mental illness, however, the evidence is often ambiguous. The jury's task can be simplified when the states rule, as the Supreme Court has upheld, that the defendant bears the burden of proof of his insanity, instead of requiring the prosecution to prove his sanity.

While we have to depend on contrasting opinions in criminal-insanity cases, I believe the margin for error could be narrowed by adoption of a system similar to that used in Norway. In that country an *impartial* team of specialists, each trained in forensic psychiatry, examines the defendant and advises the court as to its findings. These psychiatrists can be questioned during trial by either side, each of which has the option of bringing in outside experts to testify. Obviously, we could not eliminate entirely a difference of opinion between experts, but at least now there would also be an official unbiased point of view against which the jury could measure their options.

The problem with the criminal-insanity defense does not end with the trial. If a person is adjudged not responsible for the commission of a criminal act, I firmly believe commitment to a mental hospital and placement under psychiatric treatment should be *mandatory*. At present, in a judgment of "temporary insanity," the defendant may literally go scot-free. And the public might be surprised to know how little therapy is currently given those adjudged criminally insane and hospitalized. If such a person is sick, he should be treated, not just warehoused.

In addition, it appears only reasonable to me that after his release from a mental hospital the offender should be supervised by a parole board, at least one member of which ought to be a well-trained psychiatrist. We have a right to know that the former inmates of the criminal-insanity wards are being at least as carefully monitored as those paroled from prison.

Law and psychiatry are joined in an uneasy partnership in our society. As much as we want to temper justice with humanity, we also want to be protected from the Gary Trapnells and John Hinckleys who have managed to slip through the cracks in our legal system. The Constitution doesn't guarantee a perfect trial, but it does promise a fair one. That fairness must extend to both the defendant and the rest of us.

There is no foolproof method of ferreting out each and every malingerer; nevertheless, the insanity defense must be retained. Abolishing the concept of insanity from the law would be the same as depriving the individual—even when psychotic—of the God-given right to be a human being.

SOURCES

1 Life v. Death

Quote regarding Wayne Lonergan from New York *Journal American*, February 20, 1944; interviews with Lonergan, February 1944; *The New York Times*, March 23, 1944; *New York Post*, February 28, 1944.

2 The Leopold-Loeb Murder Case

Interviews with Nathan Leopold, 1941; study of his prison records; communications with Illinois Parole Board and Nathan Leopold's lawyer Elmer Gertz of Chicago, Illinois; correspondence and interviews with Leopold in 1961; *Life plus 99 Years* by Nathan Leopold, New York: Doubleday, 1958.

3 Self-Execution Through Murder

Interviews with Harvey at Sing Sing Prison, 1948–1950; court records; conferences with Dr. Bernard Diamond, 1958.

DAVID ABRAHAMSEN, M.D.

4 The Nicest Guy in Baltimore

Interviews with Frank Newell III, 1957; interviews with and notes by Robert Jett Van Horn, 1957; hospital records of his sister, Mona Lawson; police reports; Van Horn's notes; autopsy report on Mrs. Van Horn, June 3, 1957.

5 Can Forty Psychiatrists Be Wrong?

Interviews with Garrett Brock Trapnell, 1972; voluminous psychiatric-psychological reports from hospitals throughout the United States and Canada—e.g., Spring Grove Hospital, Maryland; Jackson Memorial Hospital, Florida; South Florida State Hospital; Clifton T. Perkins State Hospital, Maryland; Dodge Memorial Hospital, Florida; Austin State Hospital, Texas; Pinell Institute, Montreal, Canada; Psychiatric Division, Bellevue Hospital, New York; Kings County Hospital, Brooklyn, New York. Taped interview of Trapnell by True magazine reporter, 1971; Dr. James M. Craven's study of Trapnell under sodium amytal (truth serum); interviews with Trapnell, 1972; interviews with Assistant Commissioner of Crime, Nassau, Bahamas, April 1973.

6 Unmasking Son of Sam

Interviews with David Berkowitz, September, October 1977 at Psychiatric Division, Kings County Hospital, and in April 1978; hospital records from Kings County and school records from kindergarten through high school in New York City; military records; interviews with friends, neighbors, acquaintances, co-workers, family members, relatives; interviews with and letters from David Berkowitz in Attica and Dannemora prisons, 1979–1982; description of murders in David Berkowitz letter No. 70, November 18, 1979.

7 The Tormented Teenager

Psychiatric sessions with "Jack Casin"; interviews of parents and lawyer; police, hospital, school and court records. Freud, S: Psychoanalysis and the Ascertaining of Truth in Courts of Law, *Collected Papers*, Vol. 2. London: Lund Humphries, 1924, p. 18.

8 Profile of an Assassin

David Abrahamsen: "A Study of Lee Harvey Oswald: Psychological Capability of Murder," *Bulletin of the New York Academy of Medicine*, Second Series, Vol. 43, No. 10, October 1967, pp. 861–888. Gabriel G. Namas: "Hashish in Islam (9th to 18th Century)," *Bulletin of the New York Academy of Medicine*, Second Series, Vol. 58, No. 9, December 1982, p. 814. For a description of Marguerite Oswald's behavior and character, see Hearings before the President's Commission on the Assassination of President Kennedy, Vol. 1, p.145; Vol. 8, pp. 47, 98, 99, 254; *The New York Times*, September 28, 1964, p. 39A. For a description of the Oswalds' home life see Hearings, Vol. 1, p. 33. Private communications with Donald Jackson in connection with his writing on "The Evolution of an Assassin," a proposed article for *Life* magazine in 1964. Lee Harvey Oswald: "Historic Diary," *Life*, July 10, 1964.

9 Of Mind and Madness

Interviews at Bellevue Hospital with George Metesky; articles from *The New York Times* November 1940 to December 1973, when Metesky was released from Creedmoor State Hospital, New York. David Abrahamsen: "Insanity in Criminal Behavior," *New York Times* Op-Ed page, July 8, 1973. David Abrahamsen: *The Psychology of Crime*, New York: Columbia University Press, 1960.

INDEX